Praise for *Life, Happiness ... &*

Medical & support profession

It is a profoundly honest and simple manual. It will help p—
their families, their workmates and their therapists.
Dr Chris Atkinson MD, medical director, Cancer Society of NZ

I heartily recommend this sensitive, practical and life-
affirming guide to dealing with the complexities and
uncertainties of cancer. *Dr Roger Booth PhD, associate professor in
immunology and health psychology, University of Auckland*

This has proved such a valuable tool for all our cancer
patients, not just those living with lymphoma. We constantly
have to increase stocks in our lending library to meet demand
and having read it, I'm not surprised! *Pru Etcheverry,
executive director, Leukaemia & Blood Foundation of NZ*

This is a wonderful resource for patients, families and health care
professionals, and we will certainly recommend it to people.
*Merridee Sargent, national breast health educator,
NZ Breast Cancer Foundation*

… This is a book that I believe can make a real difference in the
lives of cancer patients from all walks of life, and one that I would
certainly recommend to patients to incorporate as part of their
recovery process. *Susan Adams, oncology educator, Queensland*

I highly recommend Phil's book … his beautifully written way
of providing helpful information will be of great benefit to others
facing a cancer experience. *Doreen Akkerman AM,
board member, International Cancer Information Service Group;
director, Cancer Information and Support Service,
Cancer Council Victoria, Australia*

I am sure there will be many people in the future who
will be helped through their own battle by this book.
Hon Pete Hodgson, Minister of Health, 2007

It's a terrific book! It's reader-friendly, knowledgeable, and
calm yet inspirational. *Dr Jeff Kane MD. US author of 'How to
Heal' and internationally renowned cancer support group facilitator*

Book reviews:

Life, Happiness and Cancer is inspirational, and will give hope and heart to everyone who has been told the dreadful news. **Northern Advocate**

... a practical 'nip at your heels' book that motivates and inspires to get your health act together ... Kerslake leads the way through the maze of current New Zealand treatment options in a clear, uplifting reminder that our biography becomes our biology. **Warwick Roger's Best of New Zealand Books, North & South magazine**

... Treading on delicate territory, he is never presumptuous, always positive ... Friends who have lived through cancer recommend this book. What higher praise could there be? **Rachel McAlpine in Upfront – Breast Cancer Network NZ**

It will enhance your ability to cope, enhance your tolerance, stimulate your body's natural healing mechanisms to function better and help you develop and maintain a viewpoint to keep you positive. **Healthy Options magazine**

For once the book promo doesn't exaggerate. Phil Kerslake really is the consummate cancer survivor ... the Cancer Society supports the book; as well it might as it is an important source of support measures for Kiwi cancer patients and their families ... Kerslake's work deserves to be a bestseller. **Wanganui Chronicle**

This is a fascinating area of research ... The book is largely about how to achieve happiness and peace despite one's health or situation, and he describes many practical methods of achieving this ... **Dr Leo Revell MD, Waikato Times**

... a book heavy with positive counsel and from-the-heart guidance ... Phil's words will bestow both important information and resilient affirmations for your circumstances. **Pink magazine**

If anyone were ever qualified to coach others on how to survive cancer, it would be Phil ... **Dominion Post**

Cancer survivors say:

I have gained great inspiration from your book. I hope that others get the chance to read it early on in their treatment plan. *Chris Stewart, Auckland*

Upon my diagnosis I knew that I was facing a psychological battle as much as a physical one... Your book was *the only one* I needed. I no longer stoop like a victim. I am incredibly optimistic about the future and shall remain eternally grateful to you for writing such a wonderful book. *Lorna Johnson, Timaru*

I am writing to thank you for that godsend of a book you wrote *Life, Happiness ... & Cancer*. It has reiterated many of my own life survival skills which I have learned through various battles and will lead me to develop more; for this I thank you. *Trevor Morrison, Napier*

Every page, every word, every sentence, I get something out of. Thanks again — you give us all massive hope. *Yvonne Robb Beaufoy, Gisborne*

I have found your book to be so encouraging and easy to read with down-to-earth practical advice ... it has really helped me to understand and cope with this illness as I'm sure it will help many others. *Shonamarie O'Brien, Tauranga*

It is a book that I will always keep with me so that I can use it as a reference and a reminder ... Thank you for taking the time to write it, and giving so much of yourself away to others like myself. *Martin Bailey, Coromandel*

Thanks deeply for your book *Life, Happiness ... & Cancer*. It has been so helpful for me, and other people facing cancer. *Rosemary Christiansen, Waikanae*

Your book gives the reader a huge range of choices, but above all it's such a relief to straight away know that you've been there (many times too!). No one understands like you do. *Lynda Going, Tutukaka*

Life, Happiness ...
& Cancer

Survive with action and attitude!

Phil Kerslake

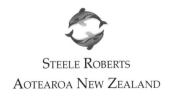

STEELE ROBERTS
AOTEAROA NEW ZEALAND

Disclaimer

The author and publisher do not take responsibility for any possible consequences of adopting the support measures recommended in this book. While the methods have provided significant benefit to many people including the author, this book is informational only and should not be considered as a substitute for consultation with an appropriately qualified and licensed medical doctor. Any attempt to diagnose and treat cancer should come under the direction of a physician. The author is not himself a medical doctor and does not purport to offer medical advice, make diagnoses, prescribe remedies for medical conditions or substitute for medical consultation.

National Library of New Zealand Cataloguing-in-Publication Data
Kerslake, Phil, 1959-
Life, happiness— & cancer : survive with action and attitude / Phil Kerslake.
Includes bibliographical references and index.
ISBN 1-877338-87-7
1. Cancer—Patients—New Zealand. 2. Cancer—Psychological aspects. I. Title.
362.196994—dc 22

Revised third printing 2009

STEELE ROBERTS PUBLISHERS, Box 9321 Wellington New Zealand
info@SteeleRoberts.co.nz • www.SteeleRoberts.co.nz

to Gillian, my best friend, my wife, my partner for life —
and our sons Rhys and Matthew, who bring us so much joy.

Contents

.

.

.

Foreword

Living with cancer is a journey. So is life … a journey to savour and enjoy. Phil Kerslake's narrative, his diary of survivorship, is a manual of how to grab life by the throat and live it, and in so doing, cussedly live with cancer.

Phil's cancer journey embraces more than 25 years, the same era that I have worked as an oncologist. Over that time patients and therapists have grown to communicate better, to learn from each other. In an era that encompasses some of the greatest scientific discoveries of over two millennia, where we now know that humans have 70% of the same genome as fruit flies, we have rediscovered the importance of self-discovery in the fight against many chronic illnesses. It is somewhat humbling to be reminded in this little but profound book, that discovering oneself will enable individuals with cancer, their whānau, and their communities to cope better and to demystify a group of illnesses that are often no more frightening or difficult to cope with than diabetes, asthma or motor neurone disease.

This approach exactly mimics the Māori concept of Whānau Ora.

Phil's book, as he challenges us, can and should be read in its entirety and then delved into in sections. Rereading enhances and deepens the understanding. It is a profoundly honest and simple manual. It will help patients, their families, their workmates and their therapists.

It is quite simply a celebration of living and proves that often cancer or living with a chronic illness can be a gift. It can lead us in other directions and enhance life even though sometimes the illness will take life.

To paraphrase Nietzsche, "We can endure almost anything if there is a *why*."

Chris Atkinson MD

Clinical Associate Professor (Oncology), Christchurch School of Medicine & Health Sciences; Medical Director, Cancer Society of NZ

About the author

Phil Kerslake, a six-time cancer survivor, has won an international award for his work in cancer support. He is a strong advocate that people with cancer take an active part in developing their own treatment and recovery plans. He recommends that patients use a range of mind-body-spirit measures during and after their cancer journey to help them cope with their ordeal.

Born in Wales in 1959, Phil immigrated to Australia with his family in 1964 before moving in 1967 to New Zealand, where he has lived since. As a 15-year-old schoolboy in 1975 he discovered lumps under his arms. Diagnosed to be part of a glandular fever bout at the time, the lumps were predicted to go away, but didn't. In 1979 more rigorous tests and procedures diagnosed a stage 2, low-grade, non-Hodgkin's lymphoma — an incurable cancer of the lymphatic system. At age 19 Phil was told he had an outside chance of living ten years.

Medical professionals decided not to treat the disease at that point so Phil got on with his life, returning to Wales and travelling through the United Kingdom and Europe. But the idea of 'doing nothing' to help his survival cause didn't sit well, so he explored and experimented with alternative and complementary medicine for cancer, then in its relative infancy and virtually an underground movement.

By 1986, with the nests of lumps under his arms ever-present, Phil was experiencing excruciating lower back pain, weight loss, nausea and profuse night sweats. These symptoms worsened until in late 1987, in what seems an ironic setting — on the battlefields of Gettysburg while on holiday in the United States — he became very ill and his battle with cancer began in earnest.

Back in New Zealand, blood tests confirmed the worst. "According to these results, you should be dead," Phil's GP told him. Further tests confirmed anaemia, hypercalcaemia, renal impairment and enlarged lymph nodes under both armpits, around the aorta and widespread in

Phil's abdomen, with disease through his bone marrow and his (grossly enlarged) spleen. Assessed to have stage 4B Hodgkin's disease, Phil began his first chemotherapy.

Battles with cancer extended sporadically over the next 18 years, with good remissions, then recurrences or new cancer diagnoses. Phil contended with six separate encounters of Hodgkin's and non-Hodgkin's lymphomas, with one immediately superseding the other more than once. He endured nearly two years and several different régimes of chemotherapy (1987/88, 2003/04), radiotherapy to the chest mantle (1989) and the neck area (1994), high-dose chemotherapy followed by a stem-cell transplant (2004), and eight operations (1979/87/88/89/93, 2003/04) including the removal of his spleen (2004).

Adamant that his cancer experiences would never limit him, Phil resolved early on to make the most of his life. He married Gillian in 1998 and the couple welcomed their first son Rhys into the world on 1 July 2007, and their second, Matthew, on 22 December 2008.

After his sixth cancer battle Phil left his corporate management job to write this book, to become actively involved in international cancer support and to become a life and leadership coach and motivational speaker. He was also a television life coach on *Good Morning* through 2006, and is one of eleven cancer survivors featured in the beautiful 2007 documentary film *He Oranga He Oranga/Healing Journeys*.

Now in full remission, Phil donates his time each year to speak to thousands of people affected by cancer, and to cancer support and medical professionals, about the principles within these pages. He is regarded as an authority on the application of psychosocial support measures to help cope with the significant emotional challenges cancer creates. He also works with health care service providers to improve the quality of cancer services for patients, and with cancer support organisations to enhance their patient support offerings.

In 2007, from hundreds of international nominees, Phil won one of three Re-Building Lives Awards in Vienna, Austria, for his inspiring story of survival and for his work in cancer support.

Life, Happiness & Cancer is now in its third printing in New Zealand, with over 10,000 copies in circulation. It has just been released in Australia, and editions are in preparation or already in print in three other countries.

Acknowledgements

I owe a special debt of gratitude to the Wellington Division of the Cancer Society of New Zealand for supporting the first edition of this book in 2006, and for being a valuable resource for my recovery programmes over many years. In particular I extend heartfelt thanks to my friends Fiona Pearson, Roger Taylor, Julie Holt and Sue Corkill.

Writing this book was a great joy and privilege, and anything but a solitary experience. I was regularly in communication with people around the world to seek opinions, exchange ideas and to invite contributions. Contacting some of the world's pre-eminent experts in their fields, I was delighted and humbled by how instantly willing and selflessly generous everyone was.

I am extremely grateful to the following people who wrote contributions or allowed me to cite or draw from their published works: Dr Chris Atkinson MD, Joanna Booth, Dr Roger Booth PhD, Professor Karen M Meneses PhD, Dr Susan Jeffers PhD, Deborah Kerslake PhD, Daphne Rickson, Dr Timothy C Birdsall ND, Dr Ruth Bolletino PhD, Dr Lawrence LeShan PhD, Emeritus Professor Miles Little MD, Professor James W Pennebaker PhD, Dr Carol Ritberger PhD, Denise Robbins, Dr David Spiegel MD and Professor Lesley G Walker PhD.

I must also acknowledge the modern-day pioneers of mind-body-spirit medicine internationally who carried out and shared the important research, paving the way for me to develop my own recovery plans and eventually to write this book. They inspired me to believe, well before mind-body-spirit medicine was even remotely mainstream, that I really could influence the outcome of my so-called terminal prognosis.

There is a special place in my heart for the many, many people affected by cancer, inside and outside cancer wards and around the world who shared hopes, fears, regrets, concerns and life stories with me through the decades. I remain humbled by your courage and your humanity in the face of cancer. For those who have passed on, I honour your memory in the best way I know how — by living every day to the fullest extent possible and by carrying a torch for the immense value of psychosocial support in coping with cancer.

Love and support can be great allies against cancer. Family and friends, too many to mention here, helped sustain me when times were hard, and have made my life so much richer in times of good health.

Last but certainly not least, to my life coach Sally Angus I extend my eternal gratitude. It's been said that everyone wanting to realise their full potential needs a good coach, and Sally became mine at the point when I knew exactly what I wanted to do with my life for the first time. I never imagined how crucial having a coach — or more particularly Sally — in my corner would be to turning my dreams, aspirations and plans into reality.

Introduction

What is your present challenge?

- Are you a cancer patient seeking information and tools to help fight for your recovery?

- Are you a relative, friend or caregiver of a cancer patient wanting to support them more effectively?

- Are you a cancer survivor in remission but harbouring fears of a recurrence or having difficulty re-adjusting back in the world, wanting help to cope with cancer survival?

- Are you a cancer support professional looking to offer psychosocial support to people in your care?

I have written this book especially for cancer patients and their support teams who want to take active roles in fighting for cancer recovery. My approach differs from some other active approaches in the strong emphasis I place on working to find more meaning, purpose and fulfilment in your life, not only to enhance your quality of life but also for the stimulation this will provide to your natural healing processes.

> *My approach differs … in the strong emphasis I place on working to find more meaning, purpose and fulfilment in your life*

The effects and after-effects of cancer diagnoses have an enormous impact on virtually everyone. One in three New Zealanders will be diagnosed with cancer in their lifetime, which means few people avoid being affected by the disease at some point, as a patient, relative or friend. Many people must contend with their own diagnosis and those of family members and friends during their lives.

The big C is not a comfortable topic of conversation, nor something we want to occupy our minds, so when it suddenly confronts us as it so often does, we are left in a state of shock, terror and helplessness. *Life, Happiness … and Cancer* will help you find your way through those feelings, to learn that you do have some power over your predicament and, most importantly, that *you can choose* the way you respond to, cope with and fight against what you now face.

The concept of taking an active role to help fight for recovery from cancer has been around for decades. When I was first diagnosed with cancer way back in 1979 there were already some great books available to guide motivated patients. Ground-breaking researchers and authors such as Lawrence LeShan, Carl and Stephanie Simonton, Norman Cousins and Hans Selye wrote compelling and inspiring accounts of how to take action to enlist all our faculties to help restore physical wellbeing.

Yet despite those and other fine works that followed, most cancer patients I interact with in New Zealand, Australia, the USA and the United Kingdom to this day know little if anything about what taking an active role in cancer recovery means in practice. Conversations in cancer wards and outpatient waiting rooms have further reinforced this. So there is plenty of scope and indeed, a need, for other voices to be heard. My book is a contribution to the cause.

My point of view has developed through almost 30 years of enquiry, personal experience and experimentation. With the dubious distinction of having fought and survived six cancer diagnoses over four decades, I have had the opportunity to act as my own laboratory, trying things out and honing the methods and their application, resolving what helped and what didn't while also sharing and exchanging ideas, tools and experiences with other cancer patients and their loved ones, cancer researchers, medical professionals and mind-body-spirit enthusiasts and practitioners worldwide along the way.

From these experiences I have drawn two conclusions above all else in relation to cancer recovery:

- That recovering from cancer becomes more achievable when mind, body and soul are all truly aligned to recovery;

- That this alignment develops more readily as we begin to search within ourselves for answers to some of life's deeper questions, such as who we are and what kind of life would we really love to create for ourselves.

The philosophy behind mind-body-spirit medicine, which most would define my approach to be, differs from the predominant approach to fighting cancer today, which focuses more or less exclusively on attacking the disease aggressively in the hope that wellbeing will emerge from the embers of the assault. But what I advocate is in no way at odds with conventional treatment programmes delivered by medical professionals. Mind-body-spirit measures perfectly complement conventional treatments and in my view there is a positive recovery-promoting synergy created when the two are employed together.

most cancer patients know little about what taking an active role in cancer recovery means in practice

While I can't provide you with any assurances about the outcome of your battle with cancer, I can promise you that by regularly using the tools introduced in this book you will:

- Greatly enhance your ability to cope physically, mentally and emotionally with your cancer diagnosis, the ensuing battle and post-treatment challenges

- Enhance your tolerance to, and speed your recovery from, the primary treatments — enabling them to be of optimum effect

- Stimulate your body's natural healing mechanisms to function better, which will help establish an environment more resistant to the cancer and more receptive to the healing process

- Learn to develop and maintain a point of view that may act as a catalyst for the positive outcomes you want from the cancer battle and for quality-of-life-enhancing changes during and after cancer.

As a layperson, albeit one with uncommon experience to draw on, I have incorporated the findings of a few other people expert in their professions or with experiences which complement my message. This has also created an international flavour as my contributors come from around the world and this is appropriate given that cancer is a truly global blight.

Each chapter covers a topic that could easily be a book in itself. So I have provided only the most relevant information, advice and direction, with my own experiences woven in at times to illustrate my points. I have also aimed to provide you with a genuine self-help resource, in that you may take this book's content and act on it readily without further guidance required from me or anyone else.

the more tactics, the more enthusiasm …the more benefit you will gain

My recommendation is to read this book from cover to cover at least once and as you do so highlight, underline, circle or otherwise identify points that particularly speak to you. After your initial read-through, return to whatever chapters you wish to draw from to develop a programme that best suits you. You may choose to involve all the measures that I present or just a select group of them. As a generalisation, the more tactics you employ and the more enthusiasm and regularity you inject into the process, the more benefit you will gain from them. Passively reading *Life, Happiness … and Cancer* may make you feel a little better but it will not provide the benefits that regularly using these tools can. *It's not enough to know, you must do*!

Finally, this book should be worn like a pair of work boots, not a glass slipper — it's intended as a functional, living and breathing resource and should be bent, dog-eared and soaked with your tears by the time you leave the hospital for the last time! Take it everywhere with you, learn its content back to front and enlist its techniques and philosophies to your cause. As you do so, I will be with you in spirit, wanting the very best outcomes for you.

Part I

Put your diagnosis into perspective

1

Dealing with misconceptions

People have more misconceptions about cancer than any other disease. It has gained an aura of invincibility which gives it more power that it deserves. Many people believe a cancer diagnosis to be a death sentence, but often it's nothing of the sort. Today many people are cured, or experience long remissions during which time they can be motivated to enhance their quality of life after finding increased meaning and purpose from their encounter with mortality.

Gaining some knowledge about cancer and the experience of a cancer battle will help you cope and prevail. This chapter aims to help put some common misconceptions about cancer and the cancer experience into context, to allow you to focus on the facts, the tangibles and most importantly, your recovery.

Cancer is one name for many diseases

Cancer is not one disease. It's over 200 diseases, each with its own characteristics. For convenience they are normally grouped according to the part of the body in which the disease starts growing. It is useful to gather some information on the type of cancer you have been diagnosed with as well as the treatment options. The Cancer Society of New Zealand is a great source of ready information. Useful also are various other cancer support organisations throughout New Zealand, libraries and international cancer support sites accessed through the internet.

gain enough basic knowledge to help demystify your situation

Take some time and effort to gain enough basic knowledge to help demystify your situation. This will also help you talk with doctors with more confidence, so you'll be able to make more informed decisions when options are put to you. I will make further suggestions on this in later chapters.

The origin of many cancers is not known

Sensationalised articles in the popular press about the causes of cancer would lead you to believe that everything causes cancer and that its origins are usually well known. In fact, while cancer's behaviour is sometimes relatively well understood, its origins are more often uncertain and mostly a complete mystery.

it seems at times that we can't do anything or go anywhere without facing the risk of cancer

Around 1950, cancer was thought to be linked primarily to the ageing process and to be genetically determined. Subsequent studies have disproved this. A range of supposed causes has been put forward — it seems at times that we can't do anything or go anywhere without facing the risk of cancer; the food we eat and the air we breathe may lead to cancer. Many of these claims seem improbable, some defy common sense, others are proven without doubt. For instance, everyone knows that smoking can and often does cause lung cancer. For most cancers, though, we can only speculate on the cause. Neither the doctors nor we can ever know for certain what caused it. If you have been diagnosed with cancer, it's mostly irrelevant now anyway. Your focus needs to be on recovery.

Our immune systems routinely hunt cancer cells down and destroy them

A major misconception is that cancer cells are stronger than we are and therefore have the advantage. This is not always so. It's also wrongly assumed that cancer cells only appear in the bodies of those of us who eventually develop cancer. Again, not so. Rather than omnipotent, cancer cells can be weak and erratic. When cancer does develop, it has managed to evade or overwhelm the defence mechanisms of our immune system, which has failed to do the job it was designed for and is capable of performing.

The human immune system is one of the most complicated networks in the body. It innately knows which cells belong to us and which are foreigners. Laboratory research has proved that our immune systems can and do wipe out cancer; scientists have witnessed them killing cancer cells. Taking action to help your immune system become stronger and more effective will improve your chances of coping better with the cancer and its treatment, and may turn the recovery odds in your favour.

People will sometimes react strangely when you are diagnosed with cancer

When diagnosed with cancer, we hope everyone will rally to our cause, but this is not always the case. As you and your loved ones face unprecedented turmoil and uncertainty, some people in your circle may start to react differently to you.

It's not uncommon to be avoided and seemingly feared at times. There's a range of reasons for this. In some cases people really do fear, on some level, that your cancer might 'rub off' on them. Some parents in the United States would not let their primary school children attend classes with a teacher who had developed breast cancer. While this was clearly ignorant and ludicrous, to their minds the cancer just might have been contagious.

some people in your circle may start to react differently

Cancer conjures up quite a different set of images in people's minds than, say, heart disease. Unconsciously, heart problems suggest to others that someone has been working too hard — overdoing it and paying the socially acceptable price. Cancer is often perceived differently. No cancer is contagious but people can react as though yours is.

There's no gain in getting overly concerned or bitter about those who distance themselves. Remember that a cancer battle is a complete mystery to most people, even though so many people are affected by it. They usually have no awareness of what happens to someone once they've gone through the doors of a cancer ward. Often all they see is the after-effects of treatments: a bald head, a thinner frame, maybe a sickly complexion at times, and certainly a more pensive and concerned-looking person.

The 'you' they knew seems to have changed, and therein lies the cause of some peoples' avoidance. They simply don't know what to do or say in these changed circumstances. Seeing you face your mortality reminds them all too suddenly of theirs also. Rather than deal with these stirred feelings they adopt the very human coping mechanism of avoidance.

You might experience prejudice from your employer

Initially many employers are tolerant and flexible with staff diagnosed with cancer. After sympathy has been expressed and time passes there can be a feeling at work, which may or may not be verbalised, that you are shirking your responsibilities. Even when you continue to work, as I mostly did, you will inevitably need time for tests and treatments and you will need your employer to be flexible on work schedules and output expectations. Some managers see people undergoing treatment as a liability, and can imbue guilt and even seek to 'manage you out' of the organisation.

after sympathy has been expressed and time passes there can be a feeling at work... that you are shirking

When I was diagnosed with a cancer recurrence in 2003, my chief executive's immediate response was that it would make me a less reliable employee. He said he could not count on me to be available to attend meetings because of my condition and treatments. Later, after a long spell in hospital, he visited me at home just before I was due to return to work and left me aghast with the comment that as positive as I was, there was still no certainty that I would survive the year ahead. He cited two friends of his who had died from cancer in the previous year, and clearly he considered I would remain 'unreliable', and was hoping to encourage me not to return.

I share this experience with a warped boss to prepare you for the worst you might face, though I doubt you will experience quite such blatant discrimination. Having said that, my experience and that of the American teacher ousted from the classroom for having breast cancer, are not isolated occurrences. If at any time during your battle you believe your employer may be discriminating against you, talk to the Cancer Society about your options, or seek legal advice.

Most people are very supportive

Most people you interact with will support you. Fellow employees are often a great source of support. Educating them a little about what is going on behind the scenes can help demystify the situation, settle unease and bring you more support than you would otherwise receive. You may not have negative reactions from anyone. I have personally experienced more love, support and encouragement from family, friends, employers (with that one exception) and colleagues than I could ever have hoped for.

Most people will show genuine compassion and empathy for you. When you are clearly at a low ebb, someone will pick you up with a thoughtful act or comment. Most people *do* care and many show it. Most people who discriminate against cancer patients do so from their own deep-seated fears or an absence of empathy for what is an increasingly common occurrence in our society.

The company and support of others is important, as having a team behind you can aid your healing and recovery. When we have cancer, people we know will need encouragement and reassurance. Right or wrong, it's a fact and we need to acknowledge and deal with it.

You didn't cause your cancer

One misconception that has gained impetus in recent years is that people who get cancer somehow helped create it. Taking responsibility for being involved in your recovery is positive because it encourages you to be an active participant and enables you to feel a greater sense of control over your circumstances. It does not, however, require you to take responsibility for creating your illness and bear the burden of guilt and self-flagellation that this produces.

Ruth Bolletino is a psychotherapist in private practice in New York who specialises in working with individuals who have cancer and those closest to them. On my honeymoon with Gillian in 1998 I stopped off in New York to experience the intensive psychotherapy over several hours a day on consecutive days for which Ruth is well known. I wanted to learn to better access and express my feelings, and to develop more clarity on the life I wanted to live. Ruth took the 'did you cause your cancer?' issue to task in an article in *Advances in Mind-Body Medicine* in 2001:

> When many clients come to me with cancer, they believe that, consciously or unconsciously, they chose to cause their illness, or at least they could have prevented it. If only they had left a stressful job or relationship, they say, or had eaten more healthfully, or if they had meditated or visualized more or better or maybe if they had not felt so angry or anxious, or sought therapy sooner they would not have cancer.

> If they are not getting well they shoulder the blame for that too and see their continued illness as their failure, so that cancer becomes a punishment for what they did wrong. On top of their illness they load themselves down with the additional weight of their self-condemnation

and guilt. It is sad and frustrating to try to help people understand that they are not responsible for being ill. We do not know what causes cancer, I tell them. Apparently it's a combination of genetic, environmental and psychological factors. We do know however that thoughts and feelings cannot cause cancer. The important question is not what caused it but what we can do to work constructively with the challenge of getting well.

while there are no silver bullets yet for cancer recovery, you can work to influence your recovery

Of course there is a great deal we can do in terms of our behaviour and attitudes to change the course of cancer, just as there is much we can do to influence the course of many other kinds of events. Years of theoretical and clinical development of mind-body science leave no doubt of this. We can increase our chances of healing through the treatments we seek, and through our attitudes, beliefs, actions and expectations. However this does not mean that we cause our illnesses. We are all far too interconnected with one another and with our environment for a simplistic statement like "You create your own reality" to be true.

If you feel that you in any way caused your disease, please put this misconception aside and focus on the solutions to your current challenge with the positive knowledge that while there are no silver bullets yet for cancer recovery, you *can* work to influence your recovery.

You CAN cope and you CAN survive cancer

Even the strongest and most optimistic of us will question our ability to cope with and ultimately survive a cancer battle at some point. There is a lot of heart to be taken from the knowledge that today many cancers have high survival rates. It's also heartening to recognise that when functioning properly, our immune system has everything necessary to destroy the cancer. When cancer has evaded the immune system, medicine has some powerful weapons to help rectify the situation. Just as importantly, there are many actions you can take yourself to establish the environment that will help the medical treatments and your body in tackling the disease.

From early on, though, you will start to understand how traumatic and isolating the cancer experience can be. You will be angry, worried and depressed at times. Amidst treatments, your days will become a topsy-turvy mix of the former usual routines, familiar faces and interactions, plus a sea of new faces on top of white coats, tubes, needles, machinery, nausea, prognosis, diagnosis, disease staging, test results, treatment régimes and emotional mayhem. For some people the experience can be very short, with several months of treatments clearing the biological disease, leaving them to wonder what it meant in the context of their lives. For others, like me, cancer can result in a drawn out, on-again-off-again journey along a testing path to recovery.

Woven in are moments of elation as things begin to improve and a remission is in sight. And if you allow it, moments of humour come along to lighten your mood and soothe your concerns along the way. Once people recover from cancer they are often accepting of and even grateful for the significant life experience they have had. While it's a challenging and sometimes terrifying experience, you do learn about yourself and the value, importance and beauty of life through a cancer encounter. A focused outlook and active participation in the recovery process may help significantly in getting from a diseased state to remission, and this is the focus of chapter 2.

2

Point of view

Anti-cancer literature is full of jargon and clichés about our mind's ability to help our bodies recover. When I was first diagnosed with cancer I had many questions I wanted answered and you will likely be the same. In this chapter I introduce key concepts around mind-body-spirit medicine and I clarify some terminology you will have heard mentioned. I also show you that mind-body-spirit medicine is a powerful catalyst for cancer recovery.

Fatalism be damned!

A fatalist believes their destiny is pre-determined and they can do nothing to alter its course. If diagnosed with cancer, at most they would put themselves in the hands of oncologists and let fate take its course. I am not a fatalist. I believe that the way we think and respond to life and its challenges can influence our happiness and ultimately our health. I believe that we can and should take action to support our cancer recovery, allowing the oncologists to do their work while we do ours. I am an advocate of complementary medicine in general and mind-body-spirit medicine in particular.

we should take action to support our cancer recovery, allowing the oncologists to do their work while we do ours

When people consider the mind-body-spirit connection, the terms *mind* and *spirit* can be misinterpreted. For instance, *mind* is used variously to describe personality traits such as attitude, emotional tendency and expression; thought patterns and processes; and way of seeing the world. In this chapter and the rest of the book, therefore, I prefer the term *point of view*, which embraces all these factors.

The term *spirit* is ambiguous, often being interpreted to mean religious spirituality. Your spirituality is the way you find meaning, purpose, hope, comfort and inner peace in your life. It can come from artistic expression or from being in touch with nature as readily as it can come from religious conviction. Your spirituality is what makes your heart sing, and what gives you a zest for life. The realisation and expression of your spirituality benefits your healing process, as I introduce in this chapter and expand on throughout the book.

There is science behind point of view and cancer recovery

You may not yet be aware that your point of view can impact on your immune system and physical health. The mind-body-spirit connection debate has polarised people in and around medicine for millennia. Over 2000 years ago Hippocrates, the father of western medicine, advocated that whatever happened in a person's mind affected their body. He believed that when a person kept good health, they had achieved a state of harmony within themselves and in their environment. As the science of medicine progressed, the physicians' focus narrowed in on the biology, and mainstream medicine sought to treat only the body.

optimism, active participation in recovery…and regular emotional expression contribute to a better-functioning immune system

In some quarters of science the mind-body-spirit connection retained its allure, and a number of 20th century researchers scientifically tested Hippocrates' premise as it related to cancer recovery. Pioneers in mind-body-spirit science found, over a number of decades, that cancer patients who have a strong sense of purpose and will to live tend to live longer than those whose prognosis is seemingly better but who display a greater apathy, depression and an attitude of giving up.

Since around 1990 the mind-body-spirit link has been a separate, specialist area of scientific research. Psychoneuroimmunology (PNI) has produced substantial and growing evidence that our points of view can and do influence our immune systems, with many studies echoing and amplifying the pioneers' findings that our points of view may enhance or impede cancer recovery. PNI studies have now shown that factors such as optimism, active participation in recovery, a fighting spirit, stress management, a strong self-image and self-worth, and regular emotional expression contribute to a better-functioning immune system, longer survival times and improved quality of life for cancer patients.

They have also shown that a variety of mind-body-spirit practices, such as those introduced in this book, can encourage and further develop a positive point of view.

Roger Booth is associate professor in immunology and health psychology at the University of Auckland. Dr Booth has been involved in PNI research since 1990, was previously actively involved in other immunology research, and has written and co-written numerous peer-reviewed articles on the mind-body-spirit interrelationships. He says:

> I have had an opportunity to observe from two perspectives how 'point of view' can help recovery — one is from the perspective of a research scientist interested in the relationship between psychosocial processes and immune function, and the other is as the partner of Joanna as she changed her life to survive pancreatic cancer. Over the last 10-15 years, mind-body research into cancer recovery has developed a variety of assisted self-help techniques to assess whether they affect the lives of people following cancer diagnosis and treatment.

> Cancer survivors have often been exposed to these techniques in regular (weekly or monthly) group 'psychosocial' support groups. In such groups they are guided by a trained facilitator to explore and express their thoughts and feelings about cancer through talking, writing and meditative imagery, to reflect on personal characteristics that might impede their recovery, to take stock of the things that give their lives meaning and purpose, and with the help of relaxation, meditation and self reflection, to experiment with different ways of being.

those who actively participate in support groups... report significant improvements in their quality of life

> How we think and feel affects what goes on in our bodies and, as pointed out by Professor Alastair Cunningham (an eminent researcher in this field and himself a cancer survivor), "your body is a 'soup' in which cells live and grow, and if cancer cells have been able to grow well in your body in the past, you probably want to change the constituents of your soup so that cancer cells won't continue to grow in the future." What is clear from the published studies using such approaches is that many of those who actively participate in support groups (or supportive, expressive therapy groups as they are sometimes called) report significant improvements in their quality of life compared with cancer patients who don't participate.

> Also, these people often make quite profound changes to their point of view about themselves, about cancer and about the meaning and purpose of their lives. In a controlled research context however, it's more difficult to

determine whether these groups of patients live significantly longer than comparable groups of patients who don't engage in any of these practices. Yet what is emerging from the research is that those who become most actively involved and are willing to engage in what is essentially a path of self-exploration appear to have the best chance of survival.

Having observed and participated in Joanna's path as she recovered from pancreatic cancer, I have seen first-hand the power of the processes that the mind-body research is attempting systematically to document. Following her diagnosis, Joanna approached what she had to do with enormous courage, determination, and humour. For example, I remember, as she was about to be taken into surgery to have substantial portions of her abdominal anatomy removed, she laughed and told me that she probably wouldn't have to worry about her weight any more.

I witnessed how Joanna's journey often involved times of great vulnerability as she sought to explore and change deeply engrained aspects of her views about her life and her worth. I also realised early on that I was not just an observer here but an active participant and that I had to change myself and my relationship with Joanna in order to contribute to her (and my) healing. Although Joanna's cancer served as one of the triggers, the self-exploration process for me has been extraordinarily valuable, leading to my developing ways of evaluating and understanding my own life path and dealing with many issues in a much more enriching way that I did previously. And as many cancer survivors will tell you, the process never stops; it is never complete. So the most salutary point of view is one that allows the process of open and honest self-reflection and change to continue throughout your life.

Dr Booth identifies the outcomes from the practice of mind-body-spirit measures which may help our recovery. These include:

1. Exploring and expressing our thoughts and feelings about cancer

2. Reflecting on personal characteristics that might impede our recovery

3. Taking stock of the things that give our lives meaning and purpose

4. Self-reflection and experimenting with different ways of being

His comments are valuable in helping place in context two of the most common cancer recovery clichés: what a 'right attitude' is and what 'a fighter' does to help their cause during a cancer battle. None of the factors mentioned point to a requirement to be fearless, unceasingly optimistic and positive, stoical or aggressive against the unseen enemy such as the term 'fighter' might suggest. Nor is there any implication that natural human emotions such as fear, anxiety or anger must be suppressed. Rather, exploring and expressing our thoughts and feelings is the approach recommended. These are particularly useful clarifications because cancer patients looking to develop a helpful point of view often say they are uncertain and confused about what they should do to create it, or fear that they might not have what it takes to do so.

Having a strong sense of your meaning and purpose

Exploring and expressing your spirituality is one powerful catalyst for healing. Examining the meaning and purpose of your life through self-exploration addresses the spirit part of mind-body-spirit. Self-reflection and subsequent lifestyle adjustments to accommodate your spirituality helps establish balance in your life.

many people suffering from cancer have an unrealised dream lurking beneath the surface

Eminent American research psychologist Lawrence LeShan has written that many people suffering from cancer have an unrealised dream lurking beneath the surface. He says that adding the power of this dream to other healing methods after a cancer diagnosis can help stimulate the immune system and sometimes can make the difference between life and death. Dr LeShan says that everyone has a natural way of "being, relating and creating" and that when they find it they are using themselves in the ways most fulfilling to themselves. After more than fifty years of inquiry Dr LeShan says he has observed that when people become committed to finding and then living in this new way (i.e. in accordance with what gives their lives meaning and purpose), their bodies' defences increase their functioning, and they frequently begin to respond much more positively to whatever medical treatment they are on.

In my experience, having a sense of meaning and purpose, and being in touch with your spirituality are not absolute states you either have or don't have. Almost everyone has something in their life that helps them have a sense of meaning, purpose, hope and inner peace, but many neglect this spiritual aspect for the most part. The result can be disharmony and an absence of joy, happiness and fulfilment.

People with a low sense of meaning and purpose often develop what I call *soul sickness*. They feel out of sorts, dissatisfied with their lives and unfulfilled. Prolonged soul sickness has two negative effects for a cancer patient. Physically, it can lead to a chemical imbalance in the body that may suppress their immune system and lessen tolerance to and recovery from medical treatments. Emotionally, the loss of zest for life will compromise their desire to fight for recovery.

American medical intuitive Dr Carol Ritberger presented a clear description of how and why soul sickness can develop and its effect on wellbeing in her book *What color is your personality?*:

> According to most of the personality theories, we each have within our own personality type both strengths and weaknesses that are primarily determined by the genetic neurological hard-wiring found in our personality traits. The more we function in our inherent traits (strengths), the stronger and more confident we become, the stronger our sense of reality, the more control we have over our lives, and the better equipped we are to make the choices that create the life and health we want. We are in a stronger position to take advantage of and maximise the opportunities that life sets before us.

> If we function outside our core traits and work from our underdeveloped psychological functions (weaknesses), then life loses its synchronicity. We become energetically drained, mentally confused, and experience physical discomfort. Our lives feel as if they are out of control, and we have a strong sense of being detached from life. We feel emotionally numb, and our thinking becomes fuzzy. We become mentally immobilised and chemically out of balance. These chemical imbalances create a fight-or-flight stress reaction in the physical body, and that stress response hinders our ability to think clearly to an even greater extent. As a result, we find ourselves caught up in a vicious cycle of psychological and emotional behavioural patterns that prevent us from getting where we want to go...

people's will to live after diagnosis varies markedly and can diminish during treatment

Before I spent time in cancer wards with other patients I had imagined that we all have an inherently strong will to live and a predisposition to fight for our lives. But I have found that people's will to live after diagnosis varies markedly and can diminish during treatment. Cancer treatments, the symptoms of the disease together with the mental stress and anguish can reduce your quality of life to the extent that life's appeal wanes. If you are somewhat ambivalent about your life to start with, due to being off your life path or even experiencing soul sickness, you will not develop the kind of fighting spirit that might otherwise greatly support your recovery.

Conclusions about point of view and cancer recovery

Two crucial points emerge from this chapter. Firstly, taking an active role in your recovery through participation in a range of mind-body-spirit measures will enhance your quality of life *and* your recovery prospects. Secondly, when you have a greater appreciation of your spirituality (or your own unique way of being, relating and creating) and are actually living in accordance with it, you will have a greater zest for life and so stand to fare better in your cancer battle than if you feel apathetic, despondent or helpless.

The remainder of this book is therefore written to help motivate and inspire you to take an active role, and to propose useful measures you can focus on.

3

You can cope

There will be times during your battle when you ask yourself "Can I cope?" The phrase *"You have cancer"* will have been the most disturbing, life-disrupting words ever uttered to you. The questions and confused thoughts they evoke may send you into a state of shock and, for a time, your senses may dull. Shock is a welcome temporary escape zone, but it soon makes way for fear and anger.

Confronting your mortality in the bald light of day, and especially in the cold silence of the night, will make you doubt your ability to cope. This is understandable, but remember that life was always by its very nature, limited. As the saying goes, *"None of us get out of this alive."* You already know this at an intellectual level but subconsciously you probably saw yourself as bulletproof.

I recall talking to one of my doctors in the late 1980s. I had turned a corner and my condition was improving at last after a series of treatment failures — it seemed that I was close to a remission. As I took a moment to feel some sense of relief, he brought me down to earth with the observation that I had not become immortal. The comment, though obvious, really threw me. I'd forgotten completely that I was still a person like everyone else in an uncertain world full of risks and hazards. I had been focused for so long on beating the cancer that in my mind once I'd achieved that, I was home free.

Your mortality is the last great unknown — of course you will be frightened. God knows I was. But if you make a decision to fully embrace your life from this moment on, cancer will lose some of its power over you and your fear will diminish. When you can get to the point of *really* focusing on and appreciating your life — something very few people do — coping with cancer and everything else will become easier.

Don't deny emotions, use them to your advantage

The prospect of a cancer battle will stir your emotions like never before. Don't deny your fear or anger. They are two of your most natural emotions and need to be acknowledged and expressed to provide release and to stimulate positive action. Have you heard the joke, "Men are like mascara, they run at the first sign of emotion"? As a stereotypical Welsh-Kiwi pre-metrosexual male, when I have felt fear I have usually acted stoically. When I have felt anger, I have acted calm and collected. When I have felt confusion, I have shown sureness.

My approach particularly during earlier diagnoses created an *illusion* of coping but it was not *actually* coping. I recognise now the extra pressure I put myself under and the additional stress I created for myself in the process. For you to cope 'well' after a cancer diagnosis does not mean appearing brave, calm or assured if that's not how you feel. It means acknowledging and expressing in a constructive way whatever feelings and emotions are coming to the fore. Taking positive action to support your own recovery is the best way I've found to put emotions to good use and to reduce stress and anguish.

> to cope 'well' after a diagnosis does not mean appearing brave, calm or assured if that's not how you feel

Anger is without doubt one of your most potent emotions, which can work for or against you in your bid to beat cancer. Both the inappropriate expression and the non-expression of anger can become a major problem for you and those close to you. In my experience, anger and fear combined may lead you to respond in one of three ways. First, you might become hostile and overtly aggressive. Second, you could withdraw into yourself and become non-communicative. Thirdly, you might respond as though you feel no anger or fear at all. You could act calmly, as though there is no major issue to concern yourself with. Any of these three responses may be problematic.

Why these behaviours might mean you're not coping

If you act with hostility, your demeanour changes for the worse. Your anger, created by fears, frustrations and disappointments will be taken out on others. The people closest to you will receive the brunt of your wrath and instead of the caring person you often were, you become moody and bitter.

One of the commonest concerns of people supporting you, when you respond with hostility focused outwards, is how to stop you taking your frustrations out on them. Typical statements from your spouse, partner or friends will be "He/she keeps yelling at me", "I've almost reached the end of my tether" and "How do I get the person I knew back?" Expressing anger in this way will threaten the positive relationships that give meaning to your life and that are strong allies in your fight against cancer.

If you become a withdrawn cancer patient you will retreat into yourself and it will become extremely hard to get through to you. While keeping quiet may seem a socially acceptable coping behaviour, it can be equally as torturous to people close to you. You create a similar torment as the hostile patient. Ask anyone whose partner sulks whether they would prefer the silence or an all-out argument. They'd often prefer the argument — at least it clears the air. When you withdraw due to a cancer diagnosis you are not sulking in the traditional sense. You may be in a state of denial, in a state of mild shock or in a 'why me?' phase. But the effect on those around you will be the same. It hurts when someone you love closes off from you for whatever reason. What's more, it will do you no good to bottle up your emotions.

keeping quiet may seem a socially acceptable coping behaviour [but] it can be torturous to people close to you

The serene cancer patient remains open and sociable and does not seem to become angry or frightened, ever. If this sounds like you, you will be seen as a perfect patient by your supporters and your medical team. You'll never complain, lose your temper or become emotionally distraught. You may be this way by nature or you may have suddenly made a personality transition. Either way you may ultimately become a source of extreme frustration and despair for those people who love you because you will seem completely unfazed to the point of appearing not to care about your own life.

This may be *the* worst way of dealing with your diagnosis, because anger and other strong emotions have no opportunity of being vented and otherwise expressed and managed effectively. They could create stress, distress and possibly a state of physical and psychological imbalance in your system. What's more, your apparent resignation to the disease *might* just be realised like a self-fulfilling prophecy.

Cancer patients bottle up their feelings for a number of reasons. Some believe that expressing feelings openly is undignified, embarrassing or inappropriate. Those around cancer patients sometimes react negatively when they express their emotions too. People with cancer often remark that they are prevented by friends and family from expressing their concerns and inner feelings directly. While their supporters are sympathetic during the patient's moments of sadness or helplessness, they can become uncomfortable and not be so supportive when the person expresses anger or frustration.

be prepared to confide in others

Ultimately, the expression and effective management of emotions is *crucial* for cancer patients so if you see yourself in the descriptions above, it's important that you reconsider your current coping approach and find ways to express what you need to.

Simple but effective actions:

1. Allow yourself to talk about your feelings

Whether you are behaving in a hostile way, or are withdrawn or accepting, or are experiencing a confused and frustrating combination of behaviours — talk. Be prepared to confide in others, to verbalise your feelings as best you can, and to express yourself emotionally. The person you confide in could be someone close to you who is willing to listen, or someone you have met since your diagnosis, an oncology social worker for instance. You may end up crying or laughing with them, or you might just talk. For many people the thought of expressing themselves to others is stressful in itself. If you're not naturally self-expressive, it will take real courage to open up to others but it needs to be done.

2. Read, re-read and act on the other suggestions in this book

Throughout this book, especially in Parts II and III, I introduce many other actions that can help you get in touch with and express emotions arising from your cancer diagnosis. First and foremost, join a cancer support group. This helps you with expressing your feelings, and gaining some sense of control over your recovery. You will also pick up ideas from the other group participants on how to cope. Meditation (see chapter 6) can be relaxing and therapeutic when stress and anger are present — try it. Writing down your feelings in a journal can be a great release and also stimulating to your immune system. Laughter is a healing response that combats anger by dispelling it.

3. Get physical

There are many ways to vent your anger and anguish through physical exertion. One very simple way is to take a pillow to task. Punch the living daylights out of it, or if punching is not your thing, pull and tear at it. Scream and yell into that pillow whenever you feel frustration building. In addition, you may want to take up some physical exercise which you can do safely (and mindful of your energy level). This could be cycling, jogging, walking, yoga, gardening or anything else that you enjoy that will allow you to burn off unwanted tension and anger (see also chapter 5 'Review lifestyle habits').

4. If necessary, get professional help

The act of *opening up* to someone else when emotional storms build within is powerfully therapeutic. But if it's not an easy thing for you to do, professional help may be required. A trained listener, a counsellor or psychologist may take you further and faster than you could go by yourself. At this time in your life, do whatever you feel is needed without concern for any stigma associated with your actions.

Participating in your recovery is the key to coping

Withdrawal is a common response to stressful situations, but I implore you not to withdraw. Let those who care *be there* for you too. This will help them feel needed and ease their own sense of helplessness. Everyone benefits from having people around them at this time who they care for and who care for them.

Spending too much time thinking about your predicament will increase your fear and stress, if not supplemented with action. Initiating little action of your own and placing yourself completely in the hands of others *might* get the results you want, but a completely passive role is more likely to make you feel helpless. It will seem as though you have no personal control over your recovery. It's your life, so your participation in your recovery process is crucial.

Coping with the emotional strains cancer creates is as testing as coping with the physical traumas of the cancer and its treatments. You need to recognise this just as you need to accept fear and anger as natural consequences of a cancer diagnosis.

Throughout your entire recovery ordeal and beyond, it may help if you recall this truism: *Today is all you ever had, tomorrow was always in question.* Cancer is by no means the only hurdle in your path. Life's full of them. Make the most of today to make your life as enjoyable and fulfilling as can be. Cancer *is* a life challenge, but you have faced many other difficult situations so far and you have coped. So too will you cope with this battle.

Part II

Take action
to support healing

4

Treatment choices

It is important to decide what treatment approach you will adopt to directly target the cancer. Your choice will reflect your own beliefs, your philosophy on medicine and life in general, and you'll need advice. In this chapter I introduce four models of cancer care and discuss my experience in the pros and cons of conventional and complementary/alternative medicine (CAM).

War of the treatment philosophies

Long before you were diagnosed with cancer you almost certainly knew, to some degree, of the debates and disagreement over the best approach to treating cancer. When you find yourself diagnosed with the disease, that debate becomes much more than a philosophical and academic argument to you.

The 'war' of sorts between the conventional medical fraternity and some CAM practitioners has been raging for decades. In one extremist corner the conventionalists say that all alternative therapy offerings are unadulterated quackery, and its practitioners are charlatans targeting vulnerable patients with useless and expensive placebos. In the

conventionalists say that all alternative therapy offerings are unadulterated quackery

other corner, alternative practitioners slate conventional medicine for doing more harm than good, for killing more people than it cures and for being created, promoted and distributed by motivations of consumerism and corporate greed.

Dr Timothy Birdsall, of the Cancer Treatment Centers of America, summed up the patient's position amidst this war in a speech to the Center for Mind-body Medicine conference in October 2001. He quoted one of his patients as saying it was like she was a child in the middle of a bitter custody battle, with two parents saying they love her but neither one of them talking to the other and maybe bad-mouthing each other.

it was like she was a child in the middle of a bitter custody battle, with two parents saying they love her but neither one of them talking to the other

Dr Birdsall identified that the cancer patient is left in the dilemma of trying to balance the information they're getting from their oncologist with information they may be getting from a nutritionist, herbalist or homeopath.

Neither of the two extreme positions is definitive or useful to you in your decision-making. While many practitioners are less extreme in their positions, most nevertheless remain clearly on their respective side of the fence, and getting balanced and unbiased information from either is difficult. Many cancer patients decide not to tell their oncologists about their CAM therapies to avoid fallout or criticism and I can understand that decision. When I opted to use the Iscador therapy to support conventional treatments in the late 1980s, my oncologist wrote to my CAM practitioner, also a medical doctor, criticised his methods directly and asked me why I would bother with unproven treatments.

Make your own mind up on the cancer treatment model you will follow. It's your life; it's your choice! As such I will not recommend one model but will give you information, ideas and opinion based on my experience to help you reach your own decision. There are pros and cons of both conventional and alternative treatments.

Conventional treatments – pros and cons

Conventional medicine comprises a number of treatment approaches, the most prominent being surgery, chemotherapy and radiotherapy, crudely referred to as the 'cut, poison and burn' régimes. Hormone therapies are also used for some cancers, as are biological therapies, also known as immunotherapy, biotherapy or biological response modifier therapy. There are numerous variations and different combinations of treatments dependent on factors such as the type and stage of the cancer involved.

A benefit of conventional treatments is that while there are never any guarantees about their effectiveness for a given individual, they have been clinically proven to work for other people before you.

Another is that there is ample reliable information available on the treatment proposed for you to consider. You can learn about treatments by reading material provided by your doctors, by cancer support organisations and on the internet.

Every conventional treatment has drawbacks — side-effects during treatment and potential consequences post-treatment. Radiotherapy and chemotherapy both damage normal cells and sometimes organs, and will suppress your immune system temporarily — sometimes permanently. Biological and hormone therapies can cause a number of side-effects, from mild to severe.

Some conventional treatments can also increase the likelihood of having future health problems. For instance, some radiotherapy régimes can cause subsequent damage to your lungs and increase the potential of getting heart disease later on, though these occurrences are far less likely now with new techniques used. Surgery is always a risky proposition and complications can arise downstream of operations. You don't want to be saved from the cancer today but die from the treatment after-effects tomorrow, so ask your oncologist to be open and clear about the risks of treatments proposed.

Some treatment régimes render women infertile and men sterile. Because of this, it's important, if you decide to proceed with conventional treatments, to try to preserve any family aspirations you may have for the future. Insist on taking any and all reasonable precautionary measures that are available given your

some conventional treatments can also increase the likelihood of having future health problems

particular circumstances. There are a number of options available such as the freezing and preservation of semen or eggs, and other options are opening up for women such as freezing strips of ovarian tissue, then re-implanting them after the cancer treatment is completed.

While it may seem obvious to take precautionary measures to preserve parenting potential, in the midst of a cancer encounter your decision-making can and will be clouded. Typically when you have potentially life-saving treatment opportunities in front of you, you want to be treated yesterday. At age 28 I was scheduled to have chemotherapy that was certain to make me sterile. My oncologist offered me the option of cryopreservation (freezing) of semen but I declined. I was focused only on my recovery, and having children was not on my radar at the time. Whether or not you currently see yourself as wanting children in the future, your needs and wants may change.

My decision and its consequences are not unique to me by any means. Often when cancer patients are being told about the effects and potential risks of treatments, their minds are not clear and they can miss entirely some key things being said. *Thus it always pays to have someone with you during meetings with medical people, preferably someone you trust to provide you with reality checks on your responses and decisions.* We are often prepared to take calculated risks to save our lives but it's important that we understand the risks and consequences and make fully informed, well considered decisions.

it's important that we understand the risks and consequences and make fully informed, well considered decisions

Despite the drawbacks I have outlined, conventional treatments have advanced significantly in many areas and remain your best primary treatment weapon against cancer in most instances. Earlier diagnoses, more sophisticated surgery and new generations of cancer drugs have all helped lift survival rates. Undesirable side-effects are also being controlled better now as hospitals place a much higher emphasis on preserving quality of life during treatments than they used to.

Alternative treatments – pros and cons

Alternative medicine comprises a vast array of measures and different philosophies. Most focus on lifestyle, diet, body and mind cleansing, purification and fortification. Alternative therapies can appeal because they are mostly non-invasive — they don't cut, burn or poison — and there is usually a lot of optimism from the practitioners about their offerings. In comparison to the more sombre environment of the conventional oncologists, the natural therapy encounter can be hope-engendering and uplifting.

People often gravitate to the alternative route for this reason and sometimes to avoid the fear associated with their reality. When I look at some of the times when I have approached alternative practitioners it was because I hoped I was not facing a cancer recurrence and knew that the encounter would be less frightening and more motivating than a hospital visit. In doing so, however, my avoidance behaviours could have resulted in dire or even terminal consequences. When you are having symptoms that cause you concern it always pays to take the more courageous decision and visit an oncologist.

The main shortcoming of CAM is that many of its generalist practitioners are not qualified to assess your condition accurately or to apply the most effective treatments to help you recover. During years of experimenting with CAM I have experienced a 'diagnosis' made via a crystal being dangled over my torso, acupuncture into an enlarged node in my neck (that was found by later hospital assessment to be cancerous), another practitioner feel the same lump and comment that he wasn't worried about it, and yet another practitioner diagnose an iron deficiency when hospital assessments determined a cancer recurrence.

The good news is that there *are* CAM practitioners who specialise in supporting cancer patients, have advanced qualifications and are competent in devising useful programmes to complement conventional treatments. The hard bit is in establishing the competent ones from the numerous patently hapless ones. This problem can be minimised if you rely on oncologists to advise on all diagnoses and primary treatments, and CAM practitioners are enlisted to help with the support programme. For me, the ideal would be to have both conventional and CAM practitioners working together in the same service.

> there are CAM practitioners who …have advanced qualifications and are competent in devising useful programmes to complement conventional treatments

I started my cancer battle in 1979 using an alternative régime and continued to use CAM alongside conventional medicines later on. The hospital diagnosed me as having a low-grade, poor prognosis lymphoma and proposed not to treat it at that point, taking a wait-and-see approach. Rather than just do nothing I opted to establish an alternative régime comprising diet modification and a Japanese anti-cancer vaccine.

I'll never know how much that régime helped stall the progress of the cancer. Ultimately though it was not enough and by 1986 I was becoming very sick, with many painful and acute symptoms. By the end of 1987 I was at death's door. It was at that point, when diagnosis showed advanced disease throughout my entire body, that I decided in consultation with the oncologists that conventional treatments were now essential to my survival. However, I never stopped examining and using selected CAM in conjunction with whatever conventional treatments I received.

My approach has always been to use whatever methods I considered might support my body, mind and spirit to help the conventional treatments work best. At various times, as well as mind-body-spirit measures, I have used one or more of: modified diet; high dose vitamin supplementation; alternative vaccines; replacement of all amalgam teeth fillings with composite ones; copious juices for detoxification, blood purification and immunity strengthening (wheatgrass, vegetable juices, liquid chlorophyll); acupuncture (for pain) and various anti-cancer commercial products.

my approach has always been to use whatever methods I considered might support my body, mind and spirit

For me, each of these measures played some role in assisting with my recoveries (though I hold none of them to be as potent as mind-body-spirit measures as catalysts for recovery). Before I adopted any of them, I read as much as I could from as many sources as possible (not just their promotional materials, which are extremely biased). I ensured that they wouldn't interfere with my conventional medications, resolved to believe completely in their ability to help and pressed on.

Four cancer treatment models

There are four main treatment models, though there may be variations on the themes. Each involves conventional or CAM measures or a combination of the two. The four models are: the segregated model, the gatekeeper model, the integrative model and the alternative/holistic model.

Segregated model

The most prevalent model of cancer treatment in New Zealand, this approach limits itself to conventional therapies in a one-size-fits-all philosophy. Treatment decisions are typically made solely by the oncologist with little patient input, though as the 'informed consent' issue has gained emphasis in recent years more patient consultation is taking place.

With the segregated model, more often than not the oncologist does not see the potential benefits of CAM. The patient, if even aware that these exist, is left to search out options on their own or more commonly, receive conventional treatments only. The patient who wants to explore CAM usually has to source each of its various products, services and practitioners one by one, and must resolve what they might benefit from in addition to what is available.

Increasingly though there are CAM service providers around the world who offer a wide range of CAM approaches considered useful to support cancer patients under the one roof in areas, including:

- Naturopathic medicine

- Physical therapy

- Spiritual support

- Mind-body medicine

- Biotherapy/immunology

- Nutritional support

Cancer support 'communities' provide CAM offerings in a coherent structure and often in a retreat setting. This can be advantageous if you want to explore CAM treatments. It's time-efficient and logistically a better approach to start with, while the value of interaction with others facing similar challenges and the networks you form cannot be underestimated.

the value of interaction with others facing similar challenges cannot be underestimated

Also, because the community specialises in supporting cancer patients and will have worked with hundreds or thousands before you, they should have the experience, understanding and competency for your needs that can be absent in independent, generalist CAM practitioners. The good ones will work with your conventional doctors and medications to ensure that the two approaches work synergistically and holistically towards your recovery, though conventional treatments are not provided from within the communities themselves. Some CAM communities are not-for-profit and so provide free or heavily subsidised services; others provide services at commercial rates.

Gatekeeper model

Similar to the segregated model, treatment is usually limited to conventional therapies in the one-size-fits-all approach. The difference with the gatekeeper model is that the oncologist may also offer a few

CAM options — but the oncologist controls access to these therapies, acting as a gatekeeper and relying on their own, possibly limited knowledge of the benefits of the CAM offerings.

Integrative model

For me, this is inherently the best cancer treatment model available. One organisation provides a total integrated programme under the one roof, with conventional treatments to directly target the cancer and CAM to help support symptom management, maintain physical and psychological wellbeing, establish a positive state of mind, ease anxieties and re-build hope, spirit and energy in the patient's life. Patient empowerment is emphasised, with the unique needs and wants of the patient paramount. The patient meets with both an oncologist specialising in conventional treatments and various practitioners of CAM. They are at the centre of the model, which provides for interaction and collaboration among the various conventional and CAM practitioners.

Sadly, there are only a small number of organisations whose services can be described as truly integrative and I know of none based in New Zealand. Perhaps the closest thing to an integrated cancer care model available to New Zealanders resides in the offerings of their local hospital and nearest Cancer Society of New Zealand branch. The society works closely with hospitals and endeavours to collaborate with them to ensure patients are aware of and can receive approved CAM support. In Wellington, where I have received all my conventional treatments, the Cancer Society is located across the road from the hospital and so I was easily able to access CAM options. If the society didn't favour or support an option I wanted to explore I simply went elsewhere to source it.

patient empowerment is emphasised, with the unique needs and wants of the patient paramount

If you like this treatment model but it is not locally available in the mode you would prefer, you may well opt to travel to where one is located.

Alternative/holistic model

The fourth model is adopted by people who do not wish to receive conventional treatments at all, and often by people who have been told conventional treatments can do no more for them. The alternative/holistic model involves the development of a programme of CAM to support the immune system, to otherwise bolster the patient against their cancer and to enhance their quality of life. The range of options is vast. If necessary, integrative-care service providers can also design a programme void of conventional treatments. The cancer support communities discussed above are tailor-made for the holistic model too.

Ignorance is not bliss – knowledge is power

You may have the impression that CAM options are widely known and reasonably well understood. Believe me, they're not. I have met many, many cancer patients in hospital wards, in outpatient waiting rooms and on international support group websites who had little and often no awareness of CAM options.

I have also met patients who were devastated and felt totally helpless because their oncologist had just told them nothing more could be done. One was standing in the middle of a waiting room in a state of complete paralysis and shock. When I asked her what was wrong, she said that 'they' had just told her they could do no more and she had been provided with no further advice or direction. If the conventional treatment options have been exhausted, the patient can feel completely abandoned, as though they have somehow failed and been discarded.

cancer is best attacked on multiple fronts

Even when conventional treatments are used and are working well, I believe that cancer is best attacked on multiple fronts and that making some enquiry about CAM options that *could* be beneficial is useful. Rather than following another patient's programme you could tailor one that is in line with your own needs, beliefs and values. Your instinct and intuition will guide you in the right direction — provided you are actively looking for your answers.

As you pursue your own path, some suggestions may help you make truly informed primary treatment decisions:

1. Get a robust and reliable diagnosis

In the first instance you are most likely to be referred from a general practitioner to an oncologist to determine your diagnosis. Whatever other actions you take at this point and whatever your philosophy on medicine, don't delay in getting to an oncologist to get an accurate assessment of the cancer and its stage.

2. Gather information

When you have received an accurate diagnosis, talk to the oncologist, the cancer support organisations and any other sources you choose to gain as much information on treatment options as possible.

3. Decide on treatments

Decide on the model of cancer treatment you want to pursue. Investigate the feasibility and logistics of the preferred option in terms of treatment offerings locally or further afield.

4. Use mind-body-spirit measures

Whatever model you adopt, include a programme of mind-body-spirit measures. This book provides all the measures you might need. Taking action and being resilient and adaptive are the keys to enhancing your prospects for success.

5. Don't give up — ever!

Finally and most importantly, *never give up!* If one approach proves less effective than you'd hoped, hang in there. Adjust it, add to it or change it. Seek solutions all the time and to maintain your spirits, focus on the beauty in life in the present (cancer battle accepted) and on the wonderful potential for the future. The key to my ongoing success in recovering from cancer has been my refusal to ever give up on myself. It's not a fail-safe strategy, but it's definitely the most powerful approach to surviving and to enjoying a quality life.

5

Review your lifestyle habits

Just as your point of view can affect your body, the reverse is true. Mind, body and spirit are completely interconnected and so it's important to take better care of your body when taking on cancer. Reviewing and adjusting your lifestyle habits is a sensible approach. It's a case of 'healthy body, healthy mind,' with pragmatism injected for balance. Sir Clement Freud said, "If you resolve to give up smoking, drinking and loving, you don't actually live longer; it just seems that way." A fulfilling, rich and highly rewarding life is surely more compelling than a longer but empty and dull one; what we want to achieve is a longer *and* a happier, more fulfilling life.

> *"if you resolve to give up smoking, drinking and loving, you don't actually live longer; it just seems that way"*

Some simple adjustments to your habits may enhance your prospects of a positive outcome from your cancer battle. Treatments and medications can take a toll on your body too and it's helpful if you are able to better tolerate the treatments in the first instance and recover faster from them in the second. You'll also want to maximise the chances of not developing additional health problems, including secondary cancers, when you beat this diagnosis.

Sleep

Sleep is perhaps the most underrated healing tool available when you are healthy. During a cancer battle it becomes vital, since both the disease and the treatments will create the need for healing and recovery well beyond normal requirements. Sleep is also conducive to a healthier emotional response to cancer, as it lessens the anxiety and depression that can arise from the stress associated with the diagnosis and the battle.

A 2003 study by internationally renowned psychiatrist Dr David

Spiegel of Stanford University has shown that sleep may be a weapon in the fight against cancer. The study showed that sleep problems alter the balance of at least two hormones that influence cancer cells — cortisol, which helps regulate immune system activity including the release of 'natural killer cells' that help the body fight cancer, and melatonin, which is produced by the brain during sleep and may have antioxidant properties that help prevent damage to cells that leads to cancer. People who wake up repeatedly or who work night shifts are more likely to have abnormal cortisol patterns. Dr Spiegel reported that there was a definite hormonal pattern that is affected by sleep, and that in itself can predict a more rapid progression of cancer.

try to handle stress well, by doing the things your grandmother told you to do

"The big problem for cancer patients is that they take too much on themselves and don't give enough time to help their bodies cope with the illness. They're worried about burdening their families and fulfilling their usual obligations," Dr Spiegel says. His advice is "to try to handle stress well, by doing the things your grandmother told you to do. By eating well, sleeping well and getting plenty of exercise you're helping your body cope better with the disease."

During stays in hospital, sleep becomes additionally challenging as you can be disturbed many times through the night by medication administration and regular nursing observation. These can occur every few hours when you are undergoing treatment. You may also be in pain or discomfort due to treatments, operations or the disease itself.

If you are in a room with other patients, you will also be disturbed as *they* are checked, treated and cared for. Of course, other cancer patients often have sleeping behaviours too — e.g. loud snoring — that can interfere with your normal sleeping patterns. Topping your sleep challenge off, some treatments will have a chemical affect that hinders your sleeping process, and the stress of the whole experience can play on your mind and keep you awake. There have been times when I simply could not sleep at all at night when in the hospital ward, and found myself walking alone, back and forth through the night in an attempt to tire myself out.

The solution to these sleep inhibitors can come from various avenues: ask your medical professionals what options they offer. Most commonly they will suggest medication, hospital prescribed or natural homeopathic aids. I found supplementing night-time sleep with daytime sleep to be useful when I couldn't sleep much at night, though taking into account Dr Spiegel's study this is not the ideal solution. If sleep deprivation becomes a serious problem you might seek other professional help. Hypnotherapy or counselling may help ease stress that could contribute to insomnia. Ask your medical team or your cancer support organisation for ideas and guidance until you can secure quality sleep to support your healing and recovery requirements.

Diet, nutrition and weight management

The field of nutrition is vast and complex; I could not hope to do the question of nutrition requirements to support cancer recoveries complete justice in a part of one chapter, when there are many voluminous books on the subject. I can provide you with some basic information, and direction on where you can find more.

When I was first diagnosed it seemed that anyone who said food could prevent, cause, or help cure cancer was considered a faddist. Today it's widely acknowledged that a third of cancers or more may be either initiated, promoted or could be prevented by what we ingest. According to many nutrition experts, our diets and nutritional supplementation can also have a dramatic impact on the effects of cancer and its conventional treatments.

a third of cancers may be either initiated, promoted or could be prevented by what we ingest

When looking at diet options for cancer recovery, there is so much information available and so many diverging opinions that it's hard to know if it's a goldfield or a minefield. Resolving what is right for you is not simply a case of sorting the good from the bad, it requires making decisions about who might be right and who might be wrong in an area of science that most of us are not familiar with.

A practical approach is to focus on the accepted basic principles of good nutrition with adjustments to account for your illness and treatments. Most of us are not adhering to these principles now, so adopting them provides a significant nutritional improvement that will support recovery.

The American Cancer Society provides some of the most useful and pragmatic advice available, a little of which I reproduce following

(© 2005 American Cancer Society; reprinted with permission). The ACS provides a wealth of excellent diet and nutrition information for all cancer patients and I strongly recommend you visit their website and review their information at www.cancer.org/.

American Cancer Society's benefits of good nutrition

Good nutrition is especially important for people with cancer. That is because the illness itself, as well as the treatments, may affect your appetite. Cancer and cancer treatments may also alter your body's ability to tolerate certain foods and to use nutrients.

The nutrient needs of a cancer patient vary from person to person. Your doctor, nurses and dieticians can help you identify your nutrition goals and plan strategies to help you meet them. Eating well while undergoing cancer therapy can help you to:

- Feel better

- Keep up your strength and energy

- Keep up your weight and your body's store of nutrients

- Tolerate treatment-related side-effects

- Decrease your risk of infection

- Heal and recover quickly

Eating well means eating a variety of foods that provide the nutrients you need to maintain your health while fighting cancer. These nutrients include protein, carbohydrates, fat, water, vitamins and minerals.

Protein

Protein helps to ensure growth, to repair body tissue, and to maintain a healthy immune system. Without enough protein, the body takes longer to recover from illness and has less resistance to infection. People with cancer often need more protein than usual. Following surgery, chemotherapy and radiation therapy, additional protein is usually needed to heal tissues and to help prevent infection. Good sources include lean meat, fish, poultry, dairy products, nuts, dried beans, peas and lentils, and soy foods.

Carbohydrates and fats

Carbohydrates and fats supply the body with the bulk of the calories it needs. The amount of calories each person needs depends on his or her age, size, and level of physical activity. Sources of carbohydrates include fruits, vegetables, breads, pasta, grains and cereal products, dried beans, peas, and lentils. Sources of fat include butter, margarine, oils, nuts, seeds, and the fat in meats, fish, and poultry.

Vitamins and minerals

Vitamins and minerals help ensure proper growth and development, allowing the body to use the energy (calories) supplied in foods. A person who eats a balanced diet with enough calories and protein usually gets plenty of vitamins and minerals. During cancer treatment, however, eating a balanced diet can be a challenge, particularly if side-effects are persistent. If they are, your doctor or dietitian may recommend a daily multivitamin and mineral supplement.

Water

Water and fluids are vital to health. If you don't take in enough fluids or if you are vomiting or have diarrhoea, you may dehydrate. Ask your doctor or nurse how much fluid you need each day to prevent dehydration.

Use the American Cancer Society Guidelines for Nutrition for Cancer Prevention below to help plan what to eat each day. The four points serve as a general guide for healthy people. People with cancer, however, may have increased nutritional needs. For example, your doctor or dietitian may suggest you increase the servings of specific types of food.

1. Eat five or more servings of a variety of vegetables and fruits each day.

2. Choose whole grains in preference to processed (refined) grains and sugars.

3. Limit consumption of red meats, especially those high in fat and processed.

4. Choose foods that help you maintain a healthy weight.

General tips to help eating during treatment

Cancer treatments can cause side-effects that upset your ability to eat. Like me, you might have to endure some or all of:

- Loss of appetite

- Weight loss or gain

- Sore mouth or throat

- Dry mouth

- Dental or gum problems

- Changes in taste or smell

- Nausea or vomiting

- Diarrhoea

- Constipation

- Fatigue

- Depression

These kinds of problems can create challenges to eating and to gaining the nutrients you need. This is when food supplements can be particularly useful, particularly soups, juices and nutrition-packed shakes and other beverages. Your hospital dietician can help with these.

Denise Robbins, a New Zealand cancer survivor, provides some pragmatic diet tips for cancer patients in her book *Cancer and how to live with it* (Emerald Hills Publishing, 2004):

- Eat little and often. It's much easier on your system and much less daunting than a large meal when your appetite is low.

- Make sure you eat slowly and chew your food well — it gets the saliva glands working and your stomach will find it easier to digest.

- Eat your favourite foods often and keep some tasty snacks at hand.

- Try not to eat alone — somehow it's much easier with family or friends around.

- Try foods that you can digest easily, such as eggs, soups, macaroni cheese, chicken in gravy, mashed vegetables or fruit.

- Drink plenty of fluids. Weak tea, tonic water and jelly are all good stand-bys, but add fluids with some energy value from time to time, such as milk, juice or cordial.

- Avoid greasy foods — your stomach will find them harder to digest and anyway, the fat is bad for you.

- Experiment with new foods and recipes (or, if you're not cooking, your partner or a friend might help with some new ideas).

- If you're feeling nauseous, choose foods that don't have a strong smell that can put you off your eating. Try cold meats with salads, sandwiches, jellies, yoghurt, omelettes, mild cheeses or mashed potatoes with a bit of butter.

- Try a small glass of wine or beer with your food — it can stimulate your appetite and make your food more enjoyable.

- Now is the time to consider multivitamin/mineral supplement tablets. Particularly when we're recovering from illness, our bodies need more vitamins and minerals than our diet supplies, so supplements may be beneficial, but talk it over with your doctor first.

Vitamin and mineral supplements

A debated point about cancer nutrition requirements is whether a well-constructed diet will provide enough nutrients to make vitamin and mineral supplements redundant. My personal opinion is that unless you have actively embraced a full, really well-constructed anti-cancer diet (which few people have), supplementation during a cancer battle can both be beneficial and necessary. Vitamins activate many of your body's most important metabolic processes and are essential for good health and the proper functioning of your immune system. I have used vitamin and mineral supplementation often, but only after researching and careful formulation of a programme tailored to my needs at the time.

The Cancer Treatment Centers of America (CTCA, www.cancercenter. com), an example of an integrative service provider, offers its patients a vitamin supplementation plan. An important fact to note is that the dosages of the vitamins applied to patients by CTCA are *specifically determined for the individual* by a physician after a thorough, individualised assessment.

vitamins activate many of your body's most important metabolic processes

Random, non-researched use of supplements without careful assessment and consideration of your unique needs may not help and could possibly do harm because some vitamins and minerals may reduce the effectiveness of certain treatments. I recommend you discuss supplementation plans with your oncologists before proceeding with them, to ensure they won't lessen the benefits that the treatments provide.

Juicing

The real power of juicing is that you can juice almost any vegetable, fruit or plant and create a highly nutritious, easy-to-consume drink. This can make ingesting some raw products much more palatable than if you had to eat it raw. For instance, you can blend raw potato juice in with something tastier, such as carrot juice, and enjoy the benefits of the live nutrients from the two.

My all-time favourite juice, which has helped me more than any other, has been carrot juice. I buy large bags of carrots and juice about 600mg of carrot juice to consume at a time (after chilling). This is not only extremely tasty, but it provides a range of terrific nutrients and vitamins, most notably large quantities of beta carotene — a powerful anti-oxidant.

If you don't own a juicer, buy or borrow one. You will find it very useful and even fun finding different nutritious foods to juice for yourself.

Body weight management

Obesity and being overweight are significant problems. Obesity and inactivity are linked to major cancers such as bowel, breast and prostate, according the Cancer Society of New Zealand. The American Cancer Society says that even losing 5-10% of your current weight (if weight is excessive) can offer real health benefits. If you are overweight, you could consider losing weight by reducing the amount of fat in your diet and increasing your activity, after checking with your doctor that this is appropriate given your present condition.

For many cancer patients though, preserving body mass becomes the challenge. It is important to keep a close eye on your own weight fluctuations. For various reasons, cancer and its treatments can start to waste away your body and if you don't keep a watch on it and ask your medical team to help you regain it, you can find yourself emaciated and starved of energy. This won't help you recover from the disease or tolerate the treatments. During two of my cancer battles I lost a full 20kg on each occasion. I turned the problem around with food supplementation and by eating more whether I wanted to or not. My wife Gillian helped a lot by encouraging and at times coercing me to eat when I had no appetite and was being stubborn and resisting.

losing 5-10% of your current weight (if it is excessive) can offer real health benefits

As an active survivor you need to take note of your weight and any fluctuations, and don't wait for the hospital to flag weight loss as a problem. Take the initiative, tell the staff and assert that they help you remedy the problem. Let your support team twist your arm to take in the necessary nutrition if you are off your food.

Where to seek further opinion and expertise

If you have the energy, time and interest to take diet and nutrition as far as it might go as a cancer recovery tool, you could benefit from reading about the broad points of view on the subject out there. There are a number of books available worldwide, such as:

> *Beating cancer with nutrition.* Patrick Quillan with Noreen Quillan; Nutrition Times Press, Inc, 2001

> *What to eat if you have cancer.* Daniella Chace, Maureen Keane and John Lung; Contemporary Books, 1996

> *A cancer battle plan.* Anne E Frähm with David J Frähm; Jeremy P Tarcher/Penguin, 1997

Additionally though, as you progress through the treatment process you will want to discuss your specific needs and requirements with a registered dietician, either in the hospital system or from elsewhere.

Exercise and activity

Regular mild to moderate exercise helps lymphatic flow which promotes your immune system's ability to deal more effectively with toxins and the disease. Exercise improves sleep, appetite and your sense of wellbeing. It also lessens anxiety and depression.

Cancer treatments and the disease itself can compromise your energy levels, making it harder to engage in physical activity. You may feel anything from a little less energetic than normal to being totally exhausted and barely able to walk. While you need to be careful in what you take on, taking up some exercise now to the fullest extent you can will help your recovery.

Since most of us are sedentary before we are diagnosed, the best approach is usually to start whatever you decide to do slowly and progressively, building up momentum over time. It helps a lot if you are able to find something that is not only good exercise, but is also enjoyable. Walking is one of the best activities for all age groups. It is good physical exercise, and can allow you to take the time to let your mind rest and relax (thereby helping you manage stress), or perhaps to work on the visualisation and affirmation exercises we discuss further on.

exercise improves sleep, appetite and your sense of wellbeing

If you choose walking as your activity and the weather is bad, don't put your health in jeopardy by exposing yourself to the elements. Your immune system will be low while conventional treatments are in progress. At these times consider indoor exercise at home. Stretching exercises, gentle callisthenics, or exercise with light weights will all be helpful. As a general guide, taking exercise between 30 to 60 minutes a day is recommended for as many days of the week as you can manage.

There are numerous other options such as swimming, jogging, sports, gardening, Tai chi, yoga, gym work (using weights or doing aerobics), cycling and so on. Cancer support organisations also suggest cancer patients supplement structured exercise by incorporating more activity into their normal daily routines. They suggest everyday activities such as:

• Vacuuming

• Mowing the lawn with a push mower

- Washing your car by hand

- Gardening

- Scrubbing the floors and bathtub

- Golfing

- Walking or biking to work or the shops

- Taking the stairs instead of the lifts

- Going for a walk in your lunch break

- Getting off the couch to change TV channels instead of using the remote

The hardest thing about exercise programmes is starting them. Once you get a habit formed it becomes easier. Do as much as you can while making sensible adjustments at times to account for your fluctuating energy levels. It is often a good idea too to involve your spouse, partner or a friend in the activity you choose, to help each other remain motivated and also to support you if you run out of steam at some point or find yourself a bit off that day.

Smoking

You can exercise regularly, eat five portions of fruit and vegetables a day and maintain excellent sleep habits and it will all count for little if you choose to smoke. The statistics on smoking and its contribution to cancer are horrific. Typically, one third of all cancer deaths are caused by smoking. Cigarette smoking is responsible for 85% of lung cancers in men and 75% of lung cancers in women. Those who smoke more than two packs of cigarettes a day have lung cancer mortality rates 15 – 25 times greater than non-smokers, according to one report. In addition to lung cancer, smoking has been implicated in cancers of the mouth, pharynx, oesophagus, pancreas and bladder, not to mention the other diseases such as cardiovascular disease and diabetes.

Smoking is perhaps the most preventable cause of death there is. In New Zealand, more than 1 in 4 adults smoke and around 4,500 deaths a year are attributed to tobacco smoking, accounting for 17% of all deaths not including deaths from second-hand smoke. Tobacco has a particularly adverse affect on Māori health with an estimated 31% of deaths attributable to tobacco. In Australia there are over 19,000 tobacco deaths per year; in the United Kingdom 114,000, with 42,800 of those deaths from smoking-related cancers. In the US, 435,000 people die from tobacco use each year. Cigarettes kill more Americans than alcohol, car accidents, suicide, AIDS, homicide and illegal drugs combined.

if you have been diagnosed with any form of cancer and you smoke, please stop now to give yourself a fighting chance

Enough said. The message is predictable. If you have been diagnosed with any form of cancer and you smoke, please stop now to give yourself a fighting chance. Most cancer support organisations will be able to help you find a smoking cessation programme to help you beat the addiction.

Alcohol

Drinking alcohol in moderation is usually harmless. Many of us like the odd tipple and research suggests that we are better off for it; the equivalent of a couple of glasses of wine a day or the odd beer is believed to be a good thing. However, heavy drinking can contribute to cancer of the mouth, pharynx, larynx, oesophagus and liver. Alcohol intake is also linked to cancers of the bowel and breast, although the evidence is less conclusive.

If you do like to take a drink, whether it is appropriate to drink at all for you right now depends on the medications you are on and the effect of mixing them with alcohol. At times you may feel nauseous anyway, in which case you're unlikely to want to drink alcohol. I chose to abstain from drinking alcohol while undergoing cancer treatments, to help preserve energy to fight the disease and handle the treatments.

Caffeine

For those of us for whom coffee (or in my case, lattes) are a significant pleasure in life, concern can arise about caffeine's potential to affect the course of cancer or to create further cancers. I'm pleased to report that the most reputable sources all agree that caffeine within sensible levels has no link to cancer. According to the American Cancer Society, "Available information does not suggest a recommendation against the moderate use of coffee. There is no indication that caffeine, a natural component of both coffee and tea, is a risk factor in human cancer."

The International Food Information Council Foundation comments that most experts agree that moderation and common sense are the keys for consuming caffeine-containing foods and beverages. Moderate caffeine consumption, they advise, is about 300mg daily, i.e. around three cups of coffee (or about three times more of beverages diluted of caffeine including lattes or cappuccinos). But, they say, this depends on the individual.

Two caveats to this good news, though. Caffeine can delay the onset of sleep and can also interfere with rapid eye movement (REM) sleep. Keeping in mind the need for you to get plenty of sleep as discussed earlier in the chapter, it's important to avoid caffeine close to bedtime, or at other times when you want to take some recuperative sleep. Secondly, keeping in mind the importance of avoiding too much sugar, it is a wise move to eliminate sugar from your caffeine drinks. From my experience, this is easier than you might think. It takes very little time to adjust to the absence of sugar in coffee or tea, and once you have adjusted, the drinks taste every bit as good as they did before.

the most reputable sources all agree that caffeine within sensible levels has no link to cancer

Sunbathing

Like most kids in New Zealand, I grew up basking and baking in the sun at every opportunity at one of our lovely beaches or in the back yard, with my radio alongside me. There was no greater relaxation and pleasure for me at that time. In the 1970s the concept of being sun-smart wasn't invented and we all put our lives on the line with the lengths we would go to for a great tan. Not only did we soak up as much sun as was available, we rarely used sunscreens and worse, we often oiled ourselves up to bake even more!

Those days are over, the damage is done to the Baby Boomer children and hopefully those of us who survived together with the generation X, Y and Z kids are now a lot smarter. I love the sensation of the sun on my body but the consequences are just too severe to justify the tanned look any more. Cancer societies internationally campaign to educate us on the damage that the sun can do to our bodies, particularly to us New Zealanders as our ozone layer has been compromised and the sun today has become toxic to our skin.

When you are receiving cancer treatments you often become particularly sensitive to the sun and to light in general. You will probably tend to avoid strong light and direct sunlight, and this is a good thing. Nicole Kidman has done very well with the milky look and we need to follow suit to avoid the risk of malignant melanomas on top of whatever cancer we have been diagnosed with. So cover up as you work towards your cancer recovery. The SunSmart code by the Cancer Society of New Zealand provides guidelines for protection from the sun: *slip* on a shirt and into some shade especially between 11am and 4pm when the ultraviolet rays are most fierce; *slop* on some 30+ sunscreen 15 minutes before going outdoors and reapply after physical activity, swimming and towel drying; *slap* on a hat with a brim or a cap with flaps; and *wrap* on a pair of sunglasses.

when you are receiving cancer treatments you often become particularly sensitive to the sun and to light

Your sex life

Your sexual energy may be affected with a cancer diagnosis, treatment and recovery. It is almost inevitable that a cancer battle will involve emotional and physical trauma that can alter your desire to express your sexuality or the way you want to express it. Changes that might occur will depend on the type of cancer you have, the treatments required and the way the whole experience hits you.

The most common issue is a decreased libido. While usually temp-orary, it is something that needs to be explained to your partner so they understand that it's not a problem between you. Another is that chemotherapy may be present in sperm, so it's necessary for men to use a condom if they have sex during a time when they are undergoing a course of chemo.

Treatments can have other physiological effects that can make sex difficult or impossible for a while. Everyone's experience is different — discuss your situation in the first instance with your medical team, to get a sense of how your disease and treatments might impact your sex life.

Some cancers that affect sexual organs directly — e.g. the cervix, breast, prostate, testicles, and others can have quite specific and unique impacts on sexuality compared to say lymphomas such as I have had. For that reason, and because it can be awkward to discuss sexual intimacy with others anyway, I strongly recommend that if you are affected by one of these cancers, join a cancer support group specific to your cancer type. It will be far easier for a breast cancer patient, for instance, to discuss their intimacy issues and concerns with other women experiencing similar things than in a general cancer support group. With prostate cancer patients, the disease and treatments can impact your sexuality in a temporary or permanent way, and only other prostate cancer patients will understand fully what you may be experiencing or about to go through and how you can best manage your challenges.

chemotherapy may be present in sperm so it's necessary for men to use a condom when they are receiving chemo

The key message about sexuality, though, is to not put pressure on yourself or be pressured by another to be more sexual than you are comfortable with at this time. The main thing is that you and those you love are focused on your recovery from this disease. The happier and more relaxed you are about all the decisions you will make during this process, the better you and they will cope with the experience.

6

Relax and meditate

Finding ways to relax is particularly important for you right now for three main reasons. First, the stress and shock arising from a cancer diagnosis can hamper your decision-making abilities at a time when you need to have your wits about you. Second, the pace of life and the pressure to 'keep up' in society may have contributed to unbalancing you through compounded stress *before* you were even diagnosed with cancer and this needs to be addressed. Third, the state of relaxation produces significant cancer recovery benefits as we are about to see.

A stressed state can result in a bevy of undesirable physiological and psychological effects for the cancer patient: quickened heartbeat, raised blood pressure, tension throughout the body, poor sleep, poor appetite, headaches, stomach upsets, tiredness, irritability, tearfulness, fear, regret, guilt and a compromised immune system. None of these helps achieve a recovery.

There are dozens of relaxation tools which help relieve stress and create a more relaxed state. They include meditation, massage, aromatherapy, acupuncture, Tui Na (acupressure), hypnotherapy, reflexology, biofeedback, autogenic training, yoga, tai chi, toning, qigong, Reiki, craniosacral therapy, shiatsu, labyrinth walking and progressive muscle relaxation.

I have opted to focus on three methods in this chapter, all proven stress antidotes. Selected for their absolute simplicity and their potency, the measures include two meditation techniques — the Relaxation Response and Progressive Muscle Relaxation, and what I term self-care.

Meditation – the power and the purpose

There are many different meditation techniques; all are powerful and can greatly help you cope with a cancer battle by short-circuiting the stress cycle and creating the opposite physiological effect to the fight/flight response. The meditative state is a natural one. You experience something close to it during your average day. Daydreaming can come close to the meditative state, as can the drift-off feeling when your mind loses itself for a moment. When I travel long distances on a plane or train I often go into a meditative state for extended periods of time without even consciously trying to.

Meditation is an ancient practice. It is certainly described in ancient Hindu texts and has long been a part of Buddhism, Christianity, Sufism and the Jewish mystical tradition of Kabbalah. In the 1960s Maharishi Mahesh Yogi started a resurgence of mediation in the western world when he introduced Transcendental Meditation (TM) to the Flower Power generation.

While the earliest meditation likely developed as a spiritual practice, it is most commonly used today as a secular relaxation tool. I learned TM as a teenager in the late 1970s. A retired Australian research psychologist established a TM correspondence course developed without religious or mystical associations, and was offering it to New Zealanders free of charge because he felt the practice was of value to people's health and wellbeing. After completing the course myself, learning what a powerful practice it was, I volunteered to help and worked on the courses with him for about a year after that.

the concept of taking time out at all is often something of a challenge, so the idea of 'sitting and doing nothing' can be difficult

Most meditation techniques use a focus for your attention such as a word, the flow of your breath or a candle flame. The object chosen as the focus is used to still your mind when it starts to wander.

Either or both of the techniques described in this chapter will enable your mind to reach a point of stillness or passive alertness. The concept of taking time out at all is often something of a challenge, so the idea of sitting and doing nothing — which is essentially what meditation is — can be difficult. We have filled our lives with so much busyness that our 'motors' find sitting in neutral highly challenging. But anyone can meditate successfully with dedication and practice.

When you meditate regularly you'll achieve a state of balance, clarity and relaxation in a short period of time. The ability of meditation to achieve a number of physiological and psychological benefits is not folklore or consumerist hype; hundreds of robust studies from respected international sources have now proven this to be fact.

A study reported in the *American Journal of Cardiology*, for instance, found that within a group of subjects with mild hypertension, those who participated in TM combined with Progressive Muscle Relaxation, health education, or mindfulness (a meditation technique where the focus is on awareness of the present moment), showed:

- 23% reduction in the rate of death from all causes

- 30% reduction in the rate of death from cardiovascular disease

- 49% reduction in the rate of death from cancer compared to those that didn't

Other reported benefits of meditation include:

- Sharpened alertness, increased energy and productivity

- Decreased self-criticism

- Increased objectivity

- Increased accessibility of emotions *

- Heightened self-esteem and sense of identity *

- Increased melatonin (the hormone identified as having beneficial antioxidant properties)

  * These factors are particularly important as they may help connect you to your sense of spirituality, as discussed in chapter 2. This — together with the extra energy, positivity and self-esteem that meditation creates — can further build your will to live, which can mean the difference between life and death at crucial moments during a cancer battle.

With such a range of positive effects attributed to meditation, the practice is something of a foundation measure for a mind-body-spirit approach in support of cancer recovery.

The two meditation techniques described in this chapter are the Relaxation Response, developed by Harvard physician Herbert Benson in the 1970s, and the Progressive Muscle Relaxation technique, developed by physiologist and psychologist Edmund Jacobson in the 1930s. Both are simple yet effective. The key to gaining maximum benefit from any meditation technique is to practise it regularly. Twenty minutes, twice a day is recommended, though initially people often start with 10 minutes, twice a day for a week then progress to two 20-minute sessions.

There is theoretically no limit to the amount of time you could meditate, however. Some alternative medicine practitioners suggest the more meditation, the greater the chances of cancer survival. Whether this is true or not, the numerous proven benefits in themselves justify taking the time to meditate twice a day or more through your cancer battle.

Two points of debate on meditation

Meditation can be learned perfectly well from a book without an instructor's active guidance, but some people doubt this. Meditation is an industry in itself, with some courses costing hundreds and sometimes thousands of dollars. Numerous people have benefited from the practice without an instructor on board. My view is that so-called pitfalls of meditating solo, if they exist at all, do not arise with secular meditation aimed at creating relaxation and balance.

the more meditation, the greater the chances of survival

Secondly, I don't hold to the concept that a person's word or mantra needs to be individually assigned to them by a 'skilled instructor', as some organisations will claim. While experimenting to develop the Relaxation Response, Dr Benson adopted a self-assigned mantra, the word *one*, and achieved the same physiological effects as Transcendental Meditation with its specially assigned mantras. TM *is* an effective technique, but the underlying principles creating its physiological and psychological benefits appear common to all meditation practices. And a mantra is simply a word repeated over and again as a point of focus for the meditator.

The Relaxation Response in practice

The Relaxation Response uses a word as the point of focus, so consider and decide on an appropriate word to use. It's important to use the same word over time. Then:

Find a comfortable seat. If you are in a hospital bed and can't move to a chair, adjust the bed to create a position that replicates a seating position as far as is possible. If you must lie flat you might find yourself falling asleep rather than meditating.

Ideally your location will have relative peace and privacy so you're not disturbed. If you are in hospital, find a spot that will allow you some seclusion. If you can't leave your bed, just wait for the most appropriate moments during the day when you are less likely to be disturbed.

Place your hands on your knees or by your side.

Close your eyes and begin to take deep breaths.

Continue with your slow, deep breathing for a minute or two.

Start to repeat your word in your mind. Concentrate completely but not forcefully on the word.

You will progressively feel more relaxed. When your mind begins to wander, quietly and gently return to your word.

Continue breathing slowly and deeply as you repeat your word.

When you find your mind in the still, deeper meditative state, you can cease repetition of your word. Only recommence if and when your mind becomes active again. You will then return to the full meditative state.

Enjoy the sensation of complete freedom from the world, the sense of emptiness, of heaviness, of floating perhaps.

Just experience and enjoy it, don't concentrate or try to analyse your state.

Continue for between 10 and 20 minutes.

When you feel ready, slowly open your eyes.

Rest there for a few moments and re-gather yourself.

Arise and continue with your day.

You've experienced your first meditation session!

Tips for more effective use of the Relaxation Response:

- Preferably practise on an empty, or at least not a full stomach

- Don't try too hard — it is of most benefit when it is effortless. The biggest blocks to good meditation are impatience and expectations.

- Don't battle your thoughts — they will enter your mind from time to time but they don't mean you can't meditate. Your mind is so busy as a rule that it's natural for it to resist a little when allowed the freedom to 'just be,' so relax with it and return to your word.

- Use quiet, peaceful background music if you wish, but it's equally effective without it.

- Wear earplugs or headphones to reduce extraneous noise if it becomes a problem for you.

- Don't expect every session to blow your mind. Typically, some sessions are terrifically relaxing while others feel less so. Overall the benefits accrue.

- Keep at it! It takes practice and persistence to realise the full benefits of meditation.

Progressive Muscle Relaxation (PMR) in practice

PMR is founded on the principle that mental relaxation will be a natural outcome of physical relaxation. The technique involves tensing and then relaxing various voluntary muscle groups throughout the body in an orderly sequence. PMR is believed to work because of the relationship between your muscle tension and your emotional tension. Only moderate muscle activity is involved and anyone can practise it, typically for 10 to 20 minutes, twice a day.

My sister Deborah Kerslake PhD is a London-based holistic therapist, hypnotherapist, life coach and lecturer. Her area of expertise is stress management and relaxation and meditation techniques. She describes the following approach to PMR (overleaf):

Wear loose, comfortable clothing.

Find a quiet place where you won't be disturbed.

Lie or sit in a comfortable position. All parts of your body should be comfortably supported, so a bed, couch or recliner might be best, though a chair where your feet are flat on the ground is fine.

Put on some gentle music to help you relax if you like.

Inhale and exhale slowly, deeply and rhythmically.

Preferably you will do the exercises with your eyes closed, but for the first few sessions you may need to have the order of the muscles you will shortly be working on in writing in front of you.

> Either way, before you start each session, close your eyes and enjoy the rest for a minute or two.

As with the Relaxation Response, allow thoughts to pass through your mind without resisting them, continue to breathe deeply and to relax.

Clench your hands into fists and hold them tightly for 15 seconds. As you do this, relax the rest of your body. Isolate just your fists and visualise them contracting, becoming tighter and tighter.

Then let your hands relax. On relaxing, see a golden light flowing into your entire body, making all your muscles soft and pliable.

Tense then relax the following parts of your body once each and in this order: face including your jaw and forehead; shoulders; back; stomach; pelvis; thighs; calves; feet and toes. Tense each part for 10 seconds, then relax your body for 30 seconds before going on to the next part.

> If tensing any particular muscle group is painful for any reason, skip the tensing step and concentrate just on relaxing it.

Try to feel as if a liquid wave of warmth and gentleness is flowing throughout your whole body as you relax between each clench.

Try to focus on the particular sensations that come from letting go of tension.

Repeat the technique in sequence for 10 to 20 minutes.

When you are ready to finish, stop tensing, keep your eyes closed for a short while and enjoy the rest.

Breathe in deeply, moving your fingers and toes.

Shake your hands.

Breathe in deeply again and stretch.

Open your eyes.

You've experienced your first PMR session!

Whichever meditation technique you find you prefer, establish a routine of practising it twice a day, every day, or more if you feel so inclined. Have fun with the technique and adjust it to suit your needs.

Emphasise self-care

A cancer diagnosis should make you think hard about self-care. These days many people are finding themselves the main casualty in their own battle to keep pace with 21st century life and its many demands. My own research into work/life balance has shown that between 25% and 50% of people in most organisations felt that their lives lacked a sense of balance, with work demands often seen as being the No 1 source of this imbalance. Added to that, we simply don't find or take the time to care for our own needs across other areas of our lives.

these days many people are finding themselves the main casualty in their own battle to keep pace with 21st century life

Continuing with your job through the cancer battle, if you can, has benefits in retaining a sense of normality and preserving your income; but working at the same pace as you did previously may be taking a serious risk with your health. Sometimes cancer patients actually *increase* their working pace and hours, feeling guilt and the need to compensate and 'atone' for times when they must be away for tests and treatments. I have been guilty of this behaviour at times and, on at least one occasion, damn near killed myself in the process. Please learn from my mistake. Right now is a time to pull in the reins, to put yourself and your needs first and to regain a better balance in your life.

The gift of time is the most precious thing you can give yourself and your loved ones right now. By all means continue to work if you are physically able, but establish sensible boundaries if these were not present before. Leave work at a pre-determined time. Don't work overtime and if you just don't feel up to going to work, stay in bed and have a guilt-free sleep. Always leave your weekends for yourself, your family and friends and be assertive when you need others to respect your new boundaries.

don't work overtime and if you just don't feel up to going to work, stay in bed and have a guilt-free sleep

People must be told and must accept your need to maximise your healing prospects. Receiving potentially life-saving treatments and resting to encourage your healing process must take precedence over work and all other commitments now. You need to become self-centred, whether this sits comfortably with you and others — or not. If you have a family with you they may need to pick up some of the household chores. They may need to adjust their lifestyles and routines to accommodate your needs at this time. This is not being selfish; it's being pragmatic and sensible given the circumstances. It's an important element of the process of fighting for your life.

Taking time out to relax includes your time in meditation as well as engaging in other restful and pleasurable things. You may also want to set regular times aside each week for such things as receiving massages; long, hot baths with essential lavender oils; or reading a good book, perhaps something that is inspiring, life-affirming or just a good laugh. Now is the time to turn your life's focus onto yourself, to enjoy your life even more despite your health challenge by establishing relaxation and balance strategies, and by paying attention to your own needs and wants.

7

Cancer support groups

Joining a cancer support group may be *the* most beneficial action you can take in support of your quest to survive cancer and improve your quality of life. Having interaction with and the support of others with cancer is more beneficial that you imagine.

A cancer support group is simply a forum for people affected by cancer (patients and their supporters) who gather together to share ideas, information, and moral and practical support. Groups differ in focus, approach and degree of organisation. Most are simple, unstructured meetings. Others are facilitated gatherings, structured in a certain way and with a set agenda. All are established with the intention of helping to relieve stress, improve the quality of life and to inject a wider support network into the participants' lives.

both a revelation and relief for me was to discover that you don't get pity from others in the group

People are able to express themselves in this safe environment, which helps establish all-important feelings of personal power and control. This has immeasurable value for you when you may have felt out of control to date and perhaps helpless in the face of cancer. They provide an opportunity to learn more about how to cope with, fight and beat cancer, and simply how to enjoy life more.

Because everyone in a group is personally affected by cancer there is an understanding of the fears, hopes and aspirations of people affected that you just can't get elsewhere. The chance to meet with people who understand and accept you is consoling and therapeutic. Both a revelation and relief for me was to discover that you don't get pity from others in the group when the group members and the group dynamic are right. Group members care for and support your recovery in practical and constructive ways. They accept you, warts, wigs and all.

Support groups have even been shown in studies to extend the life expectancy and enhance the recovery chances of participants. A notable study was carried out by the earlier-mentioned Dr David Spiegel of Stanford University in the late 1970s and early 1980s. Specially designed support groups were set up for women with breast cancer where participants were encouraged to express their feelings about the illness and its effect on their lives. They were also encouraged to network and form friendships amongst themselves beyond the group sessions. They visited and supported one another when things were not going well.

as an independent and private person, the picture conjured up by the term support group mortified me

The purpose of the groups was to improve *quality* of life for the participants. The emphasis was for the women to live as fully as possible; to improve their communication with doctors and family members; to face and overcome fears of death and dying; and to control their pain and other symptoms. Long-term follow-up of the participants, however, showed that those attending the groups lived significantly longer than those who did not attend. The social support provided and encouraged in the groups was a significant factor in how well *and* how long participants lived!

Why most people don't join cancer support groups

Most definitely there are negative preconceptions about cancer support groups. I once imagined them to be mutual moaning forums or cry-on-the-shoulder tea parties. As an independent and private person, the picture conjured up by the term *support group* mortified me. I felt that attending one might not only be potentially embarrassing (hugs from strangers and emotional scenes), it might somehow work to undermine my will and turn me into a victim. Very uncharitably, I believed that people who joined a group were not strong enough to face their battles alone. I felt, too, that attending a support group would increase the time I was viewed as 'a person with cancer.' I saw this latter prospect as reinforcing the feeling of being *abnormal* and *different* which I naturally wanted to avoid.

These were fixed and strongly held views from a man who had never participated in a cancer support group himself, but I was not alone in making blind judgements. I have heard many other cancer patients, both male and female, say that they did not want to be reminded that they were affected by cancer and that meeting with others also afflicted with cancer might do just that. I have also heard people say they didn't want to befriend others who might succumb to the disease, leaving them hurt and reminding them again of their own mortality.

My wake-up call

It took many, many years after my first diagnosis until I finally decided to attend a support group. A lump had appeared on my upper neck in late 1993 and after it was removed the biopsy revealed cancer. This time the news was relatively good — the cancer was localised, with no bone marrow involvement, and a régime of radiotherapy was carried out to clear the area of any residual disease. However I spent Christmas 1993 uncertain about my prognosis, and the stress was mounting. After so many years of having cancer hanging over my head, things were getting to me and I despaired.

The cancer continued to haunt me over the next couple of years. The *psychological cancer*, as the spectre of the disease that plays on our minds has been termed, is sometimes harder to eradicate than the physical disease.

One day while walking with Gillian through a shopping mall, I collapsed without warning. I had suddenly and briefly lost consciousness, falling away from Gillian's hand to the floor. I came to almost immediately but the room seemed to be wobbling violently like a boat in rough seas, and I couldn't get up. As I lay there, I found myself wondering if I

the psychological cancer…is sometimes harder to eradicate than the physical disease

was about to die. Maybe this was how it would be, I thought, a loss of consciousness at the feet of Gillian and then nothing?

A half-hour or so passed and slowly my equilibrium returned. I was able to get up and we walked away from the mall. For weeks afterwards, however, I experienced dizzy spells on a daily basis. The general practitioners could not work it out. I finally called the hospital on my GP's referral and unfortunately struck an oncologist with an uncommonly bad manner on a bad day. His response to my concerns over the phone was staggering: "The cancer might have gone to your brain, but it could be something else. You need to explore all other possibilities before coming in here outside of your six-monthly check. And anyway, even if your cancer has gone to your brain we couldn't get the scans until 6 or 8 weeks." Not even realising back then that the cancer could metastasise to my brain, my stress levels soared even further. I suddenly felt helpless and I knew I needed help from someone. It was then, in a state of desperation, that I considered the notion of a support group.

Initially I opted to search for a *virtual* cancer support group on the internet. I found one run out of the US dedicated to lymphoma patients, facilitated by Jeff Kane MD (whose beautiful and sage book *How to Heal* is a must-have for all people supporting cancer patients). I found some solace from the exchanges with other lymphoma patients, though in keeping with my nature soon found myself providing support to others rather than seeking it myself. Nevertheless this too was therapeutic and I discovered a lot of things while exchanging with the people on this support forum.

Not only did the people not fit the description I had imagined about support group participants, they were mostly quite the opposite — strong in themselves but somewhat vulnerable and understandably anxious, willing to both receive and share advice, and most notably for me, willing to be open and honest as I'd rarely experienced in others before. They were courageous. It takes courage to ask for help and to bare your soul to others when you feel at your most vulnerable. It was a humbling experience being involved with those people and I continued contact with them for many years.

it takes courage to ask for help and to bare your soul to others when you feel at your most vulnerable

Then one day the Cancer Society in Wellington held a support group session and I decided to attend. Despite my internet experiences I was apprehensive. This was the turning point for my views of *live* cancer support groups. The group was similar to my internet support group — strong, supportive, courageous, sharing and completely void of pretension or judgement. They also laughed a lot. The mood was anything but morbid or glum.

I realised too as I left that meeting that this had been the first occasion in my life outside of a hospital where I had sat with a group of other people who had cancer and who could relate to my experiences personally. It was like finding my own kind, people who understood aspects of my life that most people could not. I knew then what I had missed out on for years and regretted not taking the chance earlier.

I have attended other support groups on occasions since and each experience was positive and empowering. As always, each person brought their own coping approaches to the table and I found that I learned from them; we all learned from each other. As a significant fringe benefit, I gradually became more open, more giving and sharing. I believe that I became a better person for my support group attendances. When I had another diagnosis starting in late 2003, I found myself with an entirely different coping style from earlier diagnoses. This time I was able to be open to all my friends and family in the experience and I know that the reciprocated love, caring and openness made a difference for me. It may have been *the* difference in my recovery.

> *each person brought their own coping approaches to the table and I found that I learned from them*

As a postscript to my anecdote, I came to resolve the reason for my collapse in the mall. I continued to experience further symptoms and after a battery of tests over a couple of years found I was suffering from anxiety attack effects likely created by the stress of protracted cancer encounters, combined with my workaholism. As for the doctor from hell, I never got to meet him and he thankfully didn't appear on my hospital landscape again.

How to find and choose a cancer support group

You can find many good virtual cancer support groups on the internet today. If you can't get to a live group for whatever reason, they are your best option. However, I feel that live groups are more inherently personal, immediate and ultimately beneficial. My suggestion is that you actively look for and join a support group in your location as soon as possible and take your spouse or partner with you. Groups are sometimes run out of hospitals and all Cancer Society of New Zealand branches have information about the groups in their areas.

Most cancer support organisations focused on specific cancers also run groups of their own or can direct you to one (for example, the New Zealand Breast Cancer Foundation). It may be most beneficial to join one with others sharing your cancer type simply because some of the experiences shared will be more readily applicable to you. Breast cancer patients have very specific and unique physical, psychological and emotional issues to contend with, as do men afflicted with prostate cancer as I discussed earlier. However, support groups involving a mix of cancer patients can be particularly effective also.

Even the most individualistic of us cannot be islands unto ourselves. Being able to share with others brings a more settled state of mind. As a veteran multiple cancer survivor, my first advice to you is to find a cancer support group and allow the collective knowledge, dignity, strength and humanity found there to steady and ground you for your recovery process.

8

Healing as teamwork

Positive relationships have long been recognised as therapeutic. Friendships and family relationships can be rewarding and valuable, for their own sake and for their effect on your health. Research studies have found social contacts *in themselves* to have a positive influence on life expectancy, suggesting that all else being equal, the more positive social contacts you have, the longer your life will be.

Having a network of supportive people around you when cancer comes can help your cause in a number of ways, not the least being purely logistical. You need help to get about during and after treatments, and you won't necessarily be able to do all the things you could before you entered the hospital system. There may be times when your energy and strength are very low or when you are nauseous or incapacitated.

Who are your healing team members?

Cancer support groups are such valuable healing forums that they warranted a chapter of their own. Anyone else who is willing to provide support, assistance, encouragement or love is part of your healing team. Your own support network may include some or all of the following and you may have other people in your life who matter to you too.

Your spouse / significant other	Your friends
Your children	Your wider family — whānau
Cancer Society of NZ	Nurses and other hospital staff
Your doctors	Cancer social workers
Others in the community	Your pets

Your spouse/significant other

If you are fortunate and have a loving spouse or partner in your life, they can be more important than ever at this time. Their emotional, moral and practical support can bolster you against some of the fears and concerns cancer brings. More often than not they are ready, willing and able to help you in any way they can. Being *allowed* to help you is also a way for them to feel useful at this time. If they are kept at arm's length they can feel helpless. Please allow your spouse to play a meaningful part in your recovery and involve them in all major decisions about your treatments.

allow your spouse to play a meaningful part in your recovery and involve them in all major decisions

When I went through my 2003/2004 cancer battle, my wife Gillian was my number one support. She did everything from taking me to and from the hospital, to getting the necessary advice and acting on it when I was literally unable to think for myself. She dressed me before taking me to hospital on a few occasions when I was too weak to dress myself. She bullied me into going to the hospital at times when I was taking a macho 'I'll be right' stance when I was anything but. Mostly though, she was simply there for me, sitting beside my hospital bed when I woke up, providing me with anything I needed. I have watched many couples in cancer wards and have always been touched by the loving support partners provide.

Your children

If you have children, you will naturally feel inclined to protect them from the whole cancer experience. Unfortunately this sometimes results in their being left in the dark, which forces them to try to guess what is going on. When children guess, they imagine the worst. You are better to tell them, in simple terms, what you are going through. Let them know about the treatments you have chosen, and the main effects these might have on you. Let them know you might be sick, weak and tired for a while. Don't pre-judge their response when you tell them, though. Children have different coping methods to adults. For instance, they might go out and play to work things through in their minds. They may not appear upset at all. They may play up and become more disruptive than usual. Let them handle it in their way and ask for support from others periodically if you lack the strength and energy to cope with their response to your illness. Mostly though, keep communicating with them.

Other family members — *whānau*

Other family members will want to support you so it pays to keep them updated on your situation. They need to be told what you want from them. You may want a no-fuss approach, just to realise that they are there for you if you need it. Let them know that. You may want them to help you with some of your responsibilities while you are recovering. Asking for some help at this time will not be viewed as an imposition. Most people will be more than happy to help you, just as they would want you to support them if your situations were reversed.

Many ethnic groups view family in a broader context than many Pākehā are inclined to, and for them, their extended families are a terrific support group in themselves (though not an alternative to a cancer support group). Māori and Pacific Islanders in the wards often have large groups of people with them during the day, talking, laughing, making music and acting as they would in the person's home. It is a beautiful approach to help a loved one heal.

Friends

True friends are a great source of support. I was humbled and am eternally grateful for the many kind offers of help Gillian and I had. Everything from transportation to dog-sitting was offered. We rarely if ever needed to take up any of the offers but the fact that they were made left us aware that we were not alone and that we had support if it became necessary.

make efforts to keep up contact with your friends

As with your family, let your friends know something about what you are going through, and what you would like from them. You may want to talk to them about how you feel. Be clear about your needs and your friends will be supportive of you. Make efforts to keep up contact with your friends. Have someone tell them if you need time out to reflect or recover at some stage. Look after your own needs first. People will understand and anyone who doesn't is best out of your life, for the time being anyway.

Cancer Society of New Zealand

I've told you of my early reticence about support groups of any sort. It was the Wellington Division of the Cancer Society that finally got me involved in a live support group and I found a number of other great outlets through them during and after cancer battles. I was particularly blessed to have attended a writing course convened through the Society by the successful author Renée, herself a cancer survivor. Even back then I harboured plans to write this book. Renée taught me not only how to write a little better, but also that I needed to have the courage of my convictions and write without self-censorship.

the Cancer Society is a great source of information, practical advice, advocacy and support

The Cancer Society was established specifically to support people with cancer. Services are usually free for users, or provided at a nominal charge to cover costs, and include educational materials, funding for specific cancer-related programmes and invaluable social support activities that are not usually catered for by the hospital system. The Cancer Society is a great source of information, practical advice, advocacy and support. It has been a key part of my recoveries, which is why I suggest you and your support team visit your Cancer Society to start preparing for your campaign and to seek out support opportunities.

Your oncology doctors

Ah, doctors. As you likely know, doctors are the subjects of many horror stories about insensitive behaviour and sledgehammer bedside manners. While these stories are sometimes based on fact (and I've had occasional encounters of my own to forget), today they are the exception, not the rule. As your first link in the recovery chain, the relationships you develop with your doctors need to be managed and nurtured.

Because doctors still carry something of an aura of untouchable authority you might be unsure what to expect in terms of acceptable interactions. Hospitals today often have written statements about patients' rights and expectations in the hospital environment. I have my own five 'rules of engagement', expecting:

- to receive competent, proactive and informed treatments, and to perceive this is happening

- to be treated as a person who is battling cancer and not as a case, statistic or victim

- support and encouragement, not pity or condescension

- to have my unique and individual needs met in terms of communication and interaction as far as is reasonable

- that not everyone will get it right every time. I cut people slack and try to have patience to gently correct behaviours rather than jump all over anyone for what seems an insensitive action or communication.

The last rule might sound redundant, but your emotions and adrenaline have rarely run as high as they will when in the midst of a cancer battle. The circumstances are extraordinary and sensitivities are heightened, so self-restraint is sometimes called for so as not to escalate assertiveness to verbal aggression for minor indiscretions.

From my perspective as a periodic patient across four decades, and with due respect to the profession, there are an increasing number of doctors emerging with the required people skills to match their technical skills, far more so than was the case when I was first diagnosed in the 1970s. The more rounded doctors of the third millennium can help you recover while making the whole stressful experience more manageable.

Like you and I, doctors are unique individuals. They have differing philosophies of medicine and different interpretations of the Hippocratic oath. Some doctors are more open to the use of CAM therapies to support conventional treatments for instance, where others are completely closed to the idea. Some are more personable to deal with, others are matter-of-fact and to the point.

> *[doctors] have differing philosophies of medicine and different interpretations of the Hippocratic oath*

At the same time, people with cancer have varying needs from their doctors. Some people prefer a doctor to focus on their medical condition and don't really care for the friendly exchange between doctor and patient, while other people strongly desire their doctor to establish a close and more personal relationship with them. For these latter people, myself among them, the patient/doctor relationship and the trust that is established in it are as important as the treatment régimes adopted.

I have had very positive relationships with my doctors for the most part and this improved as my own communication and interpersonal skills developed. The reality is, when you treat doctors as humans and as individuals, the likelihood that they will treat you the same increases. You need to be assertive with doctors at times to ensure your own rules of engagement are honoured, that your needs are met and that you are treated as you wish. This is no different to other relationships in life, at this time or at others.

Oncology nurses and other hospital staff

As far as I am concerned, nurses are angels. Oncology nurses administer treatments to you and are in general skilled and nurturing. The compassionate care we receive from nurses eases some of our fears and stresses. Most of the dozens of nurses who have attended to me have been down-to-earth, positive and good-humoured. By their very demeanour and presence they made my daily hospital life more bearable.

You will also interact with lots of other people in the system, such as porters as you're taken around the hospital for tests and treatments, caterers and cleaners. Many people who take work in a hospital seem to have a nurturing and kindly disposition. I imagine they are drawn to the environment by a desire to help people in their own way. Even fleeting interactions where staff treat you like a person and not a case are genuine healing moments in themselves.

even fleeting inter-actions where staff treat you like a person and not a case are genuine healing moments in themselves

Cancer social workers and spiritual counsellors

Oncology social workers are a sometimes forgotten, sometimes ignored profession, which is a shame because they can provide powerful support in times of need. If you want they will listen as you talk through your concerns, and be an advocate for you in or beyond the hospital system. They will also put you in contact with other people with the type of cancer you have been diagnosed with, and with cancer support groups.

I consider myself very spiritual though I'm not religious. I enjoyed many discussions with the spiritual counsellors of various denominations who visited my ward. They never forced their beliefs on me, they simply initiated conversations. Because it's sometimes easier to talk openly with a stranger, you often open up to them as you might not to someone you know well.

Employers/co-workers

I have spoken of employers and co-workers in previous chapters. One thing I will add is the value of your spouse or partner having a supportive employer. A sometimes overlooked fact of life during a cancer battle is the additional pressures, emotional and physical, on our spouses. Gillian's employers were superb in 2003/4, keeping a close eye on her, providing the time and space for her to support me and even allowing her to use her own sick leave to tend to me.

Your pets

a pet's continued attention to you is a sign that you are still the same person

According to research, keeping pets can protect our health from threats such as heart disease and hypertension, and can even increase our life expectancy. Patting a dog or cat can undo the stress of the day and lower your blood pressure. Watching fish swimming in a tank can relax you. Contact with pets is therapeutic and some hospital programmes include the visitation of animals to patients.

I loved coming home from my stays in hospital to the wagging of our Golden Retrievers' tails. Aslan was about four and Amba a pup when I was going through my treatments in 2004. Each time I came home from a one- or two-week hospital stay Amba had doubled her size and I had to reintroduce myself as her dad. The wonder of animals is that they show you affection no matter what your state of health or your physical appearance. When you have received a cancer diagnosis, a pet's continued attention to you is a sign that you are still the same person. Their affection can help you feel 'normal' during these abnormal times and can relieve some of the stresses of the cancer battle.

Others in the community

Other people in your life will become aware of your diagnosis and many will make a contribution to your recovery directly or indirectly, overtly or subtly. People you come into contact with periodically may provide a suggestion that will help you. My dentist took a personal interest in helping my saliva glands recover after my second radiotherapy régime in 1994 (to my mouth and neck area) dried up my mouth and threatened my teeth. Each time I saw him he would also make suggestions or comments aimed at helping my overall recovery, without being intrusive. I was always touched that he cared about my wellbeing beyond my teeth.

Likewise, when I would buy vitamin and other nutritional supplements from the health store, the people serving me would often give me suggestions that went beyond their direct commercial interests. People that you have relationships with, and many who you just interact with on occasions, care about your wellbeing and their support does make a difference. Healing *is* best achieved as a team effort.

9

Active hope and faith

Hope for and faith in an outcome are irresistible forces of nature. They are cornerstones of a positive attitude which can enhance your life immeasurably, with or without illness. When treated as verbs, hope and faith help create an environment within you that is more conducive to cancer recovery. *Active* hope and faith inspire and enliven, triggering you into action. Most people recognise the value of hope and faith but many don't appreciate that they need to take action to realise the outcomes they want to occur. They 'hope' they will become better, they 'have faith' that they will recover, but they don't ask themselves the question "Okay, what can I *do* to realise these things?"

Acting on hope and faith means taking a role in establishing your overall recovery plans. Question the *what*, *why* and *when* of your treatments after educating yourself about the choices. Become a part of the solution and gain a sense of involvement and control over your recovery. Then work to help the treatments administered do what they were

become a part of the solution and gain a sense of involvement and control over your recovery

designed to do by creating the right environment in and around you. Practise the measures discussed in this book which strengthen resolve, establish clarity of thought and simply encourage you to *act*. This is itself empowering and hope-building.

There is no such thing as false hope

In medical circles there is a premise that to create 'false hope' in the mind of a patient is somehow unethical or otherwise morally wrong. I understand the point but I don't entirely hold to it. Since hope sustains life, hopelessness must have the opposite effect. Yet some doctors in their efforts to impart only 'realistic' information can in so doing err too heavily towards the pessimistic and create feelings of helplessness and hopelessness.

When first diagnosed, I was 19 years young and very suggestible. Two doctors were involved with me: one a somewhat dour man in his 30s, who responded to my direct question about life expectancy with the news I had ten years to live at most. An older, statesmanlike doctor joined us with a different message. You never really know about cancer and life expectancy, he said. Nothing was carved in stone, and I might survive much longer than ten years.

I looked to the first doctor to see his reaction and caught him rolling his eyes. The message this sent to me was *he's giving this boy false hope.* One doctor sowed a seed for me to pop my clogs before age 30, the other provided a glimmer of hope for a longer life. Believe me, I have used his words and the hope it created to my advantage over the nearly 30 years since.

When someone scoffs at another person's 'false hope,' I wonder how they would respond if their child or spouse faced similar circumstances. Would they say, *"Honey, it's pointless being hopeful."* No, of course they wouldn't. They would fight tooth and nail for a better outcome. They would do everything in their power to establish and maintain an environment of hope.

the real ethical and moral crime isn't engendering false hope; it is the act of programming people to die

The real ethical and moral crime isn't engendering false hope; it is the act of programming people to die. Taking away someone's hope is as inhumane an act as can be perpetrated and I have grown to view the words 'false hope' as seriously distasteful. At times, messages that reach you when you have cancer make little allowance for hope, and for some people this can help seal their fate on a conscious or subconscious level. There is cause for hope even when the odds or statistics are against us because there is no type of cancer which does not have some recovery rate. People often defy so-called odds to live longer and increasingly richer lives. I am one of them.

How I maintained active hope and faith

No two cancer experiences are the same. Some can be arduous and extremely taxing physically, others are relatively easy on a physical level. If you are faced with the former, including acute multiple physical symptoms consecutively or simultaneously, you can be tested to the point where recovery hopes lose their lustre and your faith is challenged. A risk emerges because if a person decides to give up on life, to let go because it no longer holds any interest for them, nature has a way of supporting them in their wish.

I have experienced both extremely arduous and comparatively easy cancer battles in the physical sense. Some produced few unpleasant symptoms and side-effects; others clobbered me. My 2003/4 episode took the heaviest toll. It serves to illustrate why hope, faith and resilience can be tested, and what can be done in these conditions to keep hope and faith alive. For a time, I was contending with these in short succession and often, simultaneously:

- Pneumonia

- Shingles

- Incessant cough

- Leg cramps

- Blocked shoulder artery, swelling my left arm to twice normal size

- Dramatic weight loss of over 20 kilograms

- Swollen feet through water retention

- Periodic dizzy spells and blurred vision episodes

- Recurring extremely high fevers (over 40°C) creating tremors, breathlessness, exhaustion and once, delirium

- Diarrhoea, interspersed with constipation

- Pain, discomfort and abdominal cramps from recent spleen removal

- Physical lethargy, making even short walks difficult

- Tubes inserted into my body to infuse and extract significant fluids

- High dose chemotherapy supported with stem cell harvesting and a transplant

- Antibiotics and infusions of other fluids

- Insomnia

- Loss of all body hair

- Income ceased, and resultant financial concerns

You can imagine that it would only take a few of these things to compromise your ability to cope as you otherwise might. So what to do? The following are ten examples of actions I took to keep hope, faith and myself alive:

1. I practised an 'attitude of gratitude' rather than asking "why me?" I just had to look around me to see that there was always someone worse off. Everyone in the ward was fighting for their lives.

2. I continually visualised my future at a point where all this was over, seeing myself well, happy and vibrant again.

3. I made every effort to communicate actively with everyone I came into contact with. Doing this encouraged them to see and respond to me as an individual, which helped me feel 'normal' and human.

4. I took *any* and *every* positive sign/result/outcome and mentally magnified it, holding it up like a trophy of war against the cancer. For instance, it was questioned whether my blood count would reach a level where I would even be a candidate for stem cell harvesting. I surprised almost everyone when my count rocketed from zero to the required level in just a few days. It was said to be doubtful whether I could be harvested for stem cells to enable my transplant. It transpired that I produced the hospital's highest ever harvest. I used these outcomes to create a feeling that I had power over the situation I was in, which really buoyed me.

5. I forced myself to eat more and more to help regain the lost weight, despite not having a strong appetite or a taste for some of the food. I also had a hospital nutritionist add special weight-gaining drinks and other meals to my menu. Steadily the weight came back on.

6. I took any opportunity between morning and evening chemotherapy sessions to break out of the hospital (with the nurse's permission) to stagger into the local shopping centre to sit at cafés, and even visit

the local zoo. This was tiring and I had to lean against the occasional lamppost, but it helped me feel like a person and not a patient for a time, and made me see I wasn't helpless.

7. I kept working on my life path audit (outlined in chapter 13) to develop a clear view of the life of my dreams — the one I planned to live after recovery. I wanted to create a life that was so irresistible to me that it would add further motivation to be victorious under these trying circumstances.

8. I would lie in my hospital bed and repeat affirmations to myself around the outcomes that I wanted to achieve.

9. I spent a lot of time planning the book you're reading now, refining earlier ideas for the structure and content. I 'saw' it in completed form and in my mind's eye imagined the thrill of seeing it in the bookstores.

10. I took time along the way to rest and recuperate between these actions, often listening to music chosen to create the mood I wanted to create at the time — either energy-boosting and invigorating, relaxing and soothing or simply feel-good music (see chapter 16, 'Raising spirits with music').

Acting in your own interests can be a challenge when the conditions are this trying. It definitely took effort, determination and the support of Gillian, my family and friends to persevere. But I created an environment for myself in which I could cope with the pressures and withstand the discomfort of the symptoms and heavy treatments that I urged the doctors to ply me with to maximise the chance of overwhelming the cancer.

My positive outcomes were a result of timely and appropriate interventions from my medical team, powerfully supported by the environment I created, and nurtured through the measures discussed in this book. I helped the doctors to help me. Does this make me or my recoveries in any way extraordinary? Not at all! I'm a normal guy who took an active approach to support his recovery, full stop. You can do the same and give yourself the best chance possible of recovering from cancer and greatly improving the quality of your life in the process.

Having a faith, and prayer

Whatever power we tap into when we engage in prayer, there is no question in my mind that it works. Prayer seems to draw a link between us and a helpful force — whether this is God in the Christian sense or a Universal God Force as some see it I can't say, but I have experienced the benefits of prayer many times. Prayer has provided me with intuitive guidance, wisdom and direction. While simply praying for a cure from cancer will not necessarily effect one, I believe prayers for guidance and support are always answered.

Some of my family and friends who have a strong religious faith prayed for my recovery and both Gillian and I were grateful for this. I'm one who's usually unwilling to do deals with the universe to have my life spared for the promise of a change in behaviour or lifestyle. It just seems to lack integrity, since such promises are usually reneged on after the fact anyway. But that doesn't stop me accepting the prayers of others when they are offered with love and gratitude, and it doesn't stop me asking the universe to support me in my recovery aspirations through my own quiet prayers.

I'm one who's usually unwilling to 'do deals' with the universe to have my life spared for the promise of a change in behaviour or lifestyle

I'm certain that prayer will help you achieve the outcomes you're after, but don't view prayer alone as sufficient active participation in your recovery. As the Christians say, *God helps those who help themselves,* so supplement prayer with action.

Take action in support of your hope, faith and recovery

Believing and hoping you will return to good health and taking steps to help your own cause will improve your chances of beating cancer. It will also help you achieve a better frame of mind to face what is before you.

You are capable of being hopeful in an active way, even in the most trying of circumstances, but it takes effort, participation in the recovery process and a strongly held desire to achieve the outcome you want. And here's a great thing: after you have found and developed life-affirming hope, faith, courage and happiness during a cancer battle, you will retain them throughout the rest of your life. If you live to be 120 you will always 'know them' in an intimate sort of way that few others will.

Hope and Faith chapter postscript —
by Professor Karen Hassey Dow

The experience of cancer provides many lasting lessons in life — the finding and sustaining of one's hope and faith are truly enriching and rewarding. As Phil states, hope and faith are not bound by religion, but spring from one's experience with a life-changing event in life. Cancer is truly a life-changing event. Cancer can also be a life-affirming event through active hope and faith. People touched by cancer find their own way that works for them. Phil has outlined ten examples of hope and faith in action, practical actions to press on toward full recovery — physically, mentally, socially and spiritually. Consider these actions and make them part of your recovery. I often hear cancer survivors tell me that cancer brings many lessons in life and I believe that having faith and sustaining hope are two very special lessons that we take with us in life's journey.

Karen Hassey Dow PhD, RN, FAAN is Professor in the School of Nursing at the University of Central Florida, US. Karen, who has one of only five endowed chairs in oncology nursing in the United States, has worked for more than 30 years to improve the care of patients with cancer.

10

Mind your language

This chapter and the next two are closely interrelated, and illustrate the importance of your language and imagination in creating and keeping a positive outlook. This chapter looks at how your own words, and the words of others, in day-to-day interactions influence how you feel about yourself and your recovery.

Words create and reinforce images of ourselves

Your choice of words can play a big part in *creating* the way you feel about who you are and what your situation is, and in *changing* the way you feel. After all, your core beliefs were formed through words. I have already talked about how people — doctors for instance — can say

words have the ability to build images which your subconscious mind accepts, more or less unchallenged

things that build or diminish your hope. They can do this because words have the ability to build images which your subconscious mind accepts, more or less unchallenged. You can literally talk yourself into a state of happiness and strength, or conversely, talk yourself into an unhappy and weak frame of mind. You can also be talked into a positive or negative state by someone else if you allow it.

To illustrate how others' negative words can affect you in ordinary interactions with or without cancer, imagine this quite common situation. You're in the office tea room making a coffee and feeling fine. A workmate joins you, smiling at first, then develops a frown: *"Are you okay?"* they ask. *"You're looking a bit off-colour. Are you sure you're okay?"* You *were* feeling okay — initially. Now you're not quite sure. You're starting to feel a little out of sorts. Maybe you should go to bed for a while? This person has led you to question yourself and your health. They have inadvertently planted a negative seed. You might well be feeling off-colour soon, just as they had suggested.

Words from the white coats that help and harm

I have always found hope-inducing comments from doctors particularly powerful. We still bestow doctors with an air of all-knowing authority, whether we mean to or not. It's built into our psyches and difficult to overcome. So at a moment when we are feeling worried and vulnerable, 'helpful' words from a doctor can be terrifically uplifting — while ill-considered, 'harmful' ones can be devastating.

Many cancer survivors can recount throwaway comments made by medical people that made them feel like victims, belittled their situation or implied they might as well give up hope. The words and their effect are always completely inadvertent, but harmful on a number of levels. Once when I was having chemotherapy, a doctor made the off-hand comment *"Don't worry, if this doesn't work, nothing will."* The comment created anxiety for me because I knew in myself that the chemotherapy wasn't working. Something else *was* going to have to do the job and he was suggesting in his comment there *was nothing* else.

The American National Coalition for Cancer Survivorship undertook a study in 1995 to look at words cancer survivors found most helpful from their doctors, and those they found most harmful. Most helpful were words that:

- were proactive and empowering

- normalised the cancer experience

- acknowledged individual differences

- conveyed hope

- reframed the problem more clearly and positively

- showed genuineness and compassion

- assured continuing support

Most harmful were words that:

- suggested lack of control over the disease

- were trite or took the form of platitudes

- compared survivors to others or to statistics

- disregarded feelings and concerns

- were cold or cynical

- indicated continuing support was conditional

- destroyed hope

Minding your own language – talking 'as if'

Without even noticing it, we all have habitual language that affects the way we feel about ourselves and our lives. How we talk about ourselves and our challenges sends messages to our subconscious, for better or worse. When we learn that our words and those of others can make a difference to how we feel, we can begin to influence words spoken to us and modify our own words to our advantage. Words can become powerful tools in helping to create our wellbeing. In choosing to reject the cancer, one of the first positive steps you can take is to avoid *victim language* of your own. This means thinking about what you say and using words that reinforce *you* as a strong person with some control over your recovery.

one of the first positive steps you can take is to avoid victim language of your own

Affirmations are a particularly effective measure to channel you from a victim mentality to an empowered mind-set — I discuss these further in chapter 12. But simply replacing negative and passive language with more positive and powerful words in daily conversation sends corresponding images to your subconscious mind.

There's a well accepted concept in self-help doctrine called 'acting as if'. Acting as if you are strong, optimistic and powerful can actually help you feel that way. 'Talking as if' can have the same benefits. When I was undergoing chemotherapy there were times when I felt unwell. There were other times when I felt pretty awful. I might have been nauseous, tired, dizzy, on an emotional rollercoaster, or a whole host of other things that cancer and chemotherapy can contribute to making you feel. But when anyone asked me how I was that day, I always tried to respond positively with a *"Great, thanks"* or *"Getting better, thanks."*

I wasn't putting on a brave face, or being some kind of martyr. I have simply found over the years that whenever I hear myself say positive things about me, I actually feel and cope better. Conversely, if I was feeling rotten and said how I felt in reality, I found that I reinforced that feeling, or even started to feel worse.

My yardstick for my frame of mind during diagnoses was often my response to *"How are you?"* I took stock one day and realised I had started to respond to that question a different way. Instead of my standard *"Great, thanks"* or similar affirming response, I found myself considering the question longer and giving more of an events and symptoms update. It occurred to me that I had started to doubt and question rather than believe implicitly in my recovery, and my optimism was being eroded further as I did so. This realisation prompted me to return to positive-speak and consequently get my recovery back on track.

Use your words for better, not worse

We often prefer to share bad news rather than good news. Bad news is somehow more interesting and newsworthy. It's also true that we like to talk in negatives at times. We like to have something to complain or gossip about. Louise Hay, best-selling author and one of the founders of the self-help movement, has said that when she had cancer she made a conscious decision to stop gossiping about other people to her friends. She surprised herself when she discovered she now had nothing to talk about! She found, like I did, that changing habitual language takes effort and work. But like me she found it of immense value in adding joy and hope to her life as well.

What you say about yourself and others will have a positive or negative impact on you. If for instance, you say *"I am weak and the cancer is strong"*, you immediately empower the cancer and disempower yourself. In a sense you hand your power to the disease. Here are some words that can empower you and their disempowering counterparts, to suggest what you might notice in your daily language and choose to modify.

Disempowering words (stop using)	Empowering words (use these!)
I'm a cancer victim	I'm fighting a cancer!
I'm helpless	I am beating this!
I don't know if I can cope	I am handling it!
I have to have chemo	I've chosen to have chemo!
I'm weak	I'm a strong person!
I'm not ...	I am and I will!
The odds are against me	Odds mean nothing. I'm an individual!
Life is tough	Life is great and getting better!

These words relate directly to the cancer diagnosis and battle, but it is worth modifying any negative words you use during this time and from here on. Rather than discussing negative things with others, turn your conversations to more positive, hopeful and optimistic things. This will help lift your mood and create optimistic feelings and expectations. It's also useful to re-phrase concerns you have at times into questions that lead to problem-solving. For instance:

Concern	Rephrased as problem-solving question
I'm scared	What can I do to help overcome my fear?
I feel awful	What actions or medications can I take to feel better in myself?
I feel my doctor is not involving me	Doctor, I'd like more involvement in the decisions that affect me, please. How can we make this happen?

Finally, the intonation and emotion you attach to words can influence how they are interpreted by your subconscious. Using an upbeat tone with the positive words helps them hit home because words uttered with emotional intensity are especially powerful.

Noticing what you say, and modifying the language when and where you feel it's appropriate in a natural and relaxed way, will help your recovery cause. Taking a position on the words you are prepared to use and not use and accept from others represents taking a position against the cancer. My life keeps getting better and better as I work to take the positive from every situation and use words to reinforce how I wish to feel.

Sometimes, especially if you're feeling less than 100% and saying to yourself that you're feeling well or better, you may suddenly think *"Who am I kidding?"* That's natural. But keep saying it often and you'll be pleasantly surprised when you actually start to feel better. I kidded myself time and time again into feeling better, stronger and healthier than I probably was at the time. I believe that *kidding myself* was a key factor in my ultimate recovery.

11

Visualise health

Visualisation is a highly effective way to help you create whatever you want in life. Also known as guided imagery, visualisation directs your imagination towards a desired condition or outcome. It's universally accepted now as a powerful tool to help create relaxation during the distressful cancer diagnosis. Clinical studies have shown the ability of positive visualisation to boost the human immune system, though not yet impact the course of a cancer.

Cancer Research UK reports a trial by Professor Leslie Walker at the University of Aberdeen involving 80 women diagnosed with breast cancer. The women had standard treatments such as chemotherapy, radio-therapy, surgery and hormone therapy. Half of them were taught relaxation techniques and guided imagery, while half were not. The guided imagery had the women picturing their immune systems trying to get rid of cancer cells or otherwise improving their health. By the end of the 37-week trial, the women practising relaxation and visualisation said they had a better quality of life during the chemotherapy; were in a more positive mood, and seemed better able to cope with their illness and treatment. Also, compared to the group not using relaxation and visualisation, they had an increase in the number of various types of white blood cells that fight disease!

using positive imagery, combined with the adoption of helpful language, can have a terrific impact on your frame of mind

I used visualisation frequently for a number of purposes during my cancer battles. There is no question in my mind that using positive imagery, combined with the adoption of helpful language, can have a terrific impact on your frame of mind and outlook for the future and therefore your recovery prospects.

Visualisation is a natural act

You already practise visualisation as a matter of course, though you probably don't realise it. When you 'see' yourself in a certain way, positive or negative, you are visualising yourself in one direction or another, for better or worse. If you see yourself as unattractive, unintelligent, unloved or unlucky, you probably helped create those outcomes or beliefs through negative self-talk and self-imaging. On the other hand if you have chosen to see yourself as intelligent, attractive, loved and lucky, you have contributed to those beliefs through positive self-talk and positive self-imaging. It's a natural process that we engage in unconsciously. What I propose is that you use positive self-talk and self-imaging to support your recovery in a conscious and deliberate way. You can use visualisation to achieve a number of different cancer recovery objectives. Those I have targeted my visualisation towards include:

- Building optimism for and belief in recovery

- Adding power to medical treatments as they are being administered

- Attacking the cancer to reduce its mass or stop its progress

Four key ways to practise visualisation:

- Self-guided

- Guided by another person

- Guided by an audio facility (tape/CD)

- Guided under hypnosis by a hypnotherapist

Self-guided visualisation – the do-it-yourself approach

With self-guided visualisation, you do it without any guide. There are three simple steps to self-guided visualisation:

- Decide what the objective of the session will be

- Establish a comfortable and relaxed state

- Convene your visualisation for about 20 minutes at a time

After deciding on the objective of your visualisation session, find a comfortable place where you won't be disturbed — hang a sign on the door if you can — and start to relax yourself. I have found that just sitting or lying in a comfortable position, away from interruption, and spending five minutes or so imagining my body relaxing, while taking deep breaths, puts me in a state receptive to the imagery.

Many people choose to establish an imaginary sanctuary for their visualisation, somewhere they will go to in their mind's eye. Some create an imaginary room — a safe place which no one can enter without their permission. They create it in their favourite colours, that they feel soothed by. Other sanctuaries might be beside a pool, an ocean, on a mountain, at a favourite park or even on a cloud. Everyone has a different concept of what they see as safe and restful, so choose what works for you.

Building optimism for and belief in recovery

While in your sanctuary and in a relaxed state, see yourself strong, powerful and in control of everything around you. See yourself smiling with contentment at the strength and vitality you have gained. Create a sense of confidence about your strength, a sense of 'knowing' that you have power without limits. Feel it flow into your body. Imagine yourself performing feats of strength with boundless energy which you can direct towards any activity you wish.

make the visualisation as completely real and alive as you can make it

An effective practice with all visualisation work is to employ every one of your senses in the process. For example, if you were visualising yourself as a weightlifter pressing great weight over your head, feel the cold bar in your hands, see the crowd watching and hear their applause. Smell liniment on your hands, taste the sweet liquid you drank just before you took the barbell, and experience the rush of elation as you achieve your objective of pressing the weight. Make the visualisation as completely real and alive as you can make it.

A powerful method that I have used to reaffirm belief in my recovery is to project myself into the future. Imagine yourself in two years, five years then ten years. See how you look, what you are doing, who is with you, where you are. See yourself well, happy, strong and motivated and feel the sense of satisfaction and fulfilment you have established in your life. This is a great chance to reaffirm the life of your dreams as discussed later in chapter 13. See yourself clearly and make links — like invisible umbilical cords, to each of your future selves. You are creating these psychic links with the future to help you *create* what you really want.

There are no limits in matters of the imagination except for those you allow, so take the chance to imagine big! As with all your visualisation exercises, it will help to create positive emotional intensity around where you go and what you do. So *really* feel how thrilling and exciting it is to meet your future selves and to know that *you will be them* in all their happiness, fulfilment and success in the passage of time.

Adding power to medical treatments as they are being administered

I often used this approach as I received chemotherapy intravenously and this is probably its best application, though it can be used as any other treatment is being administered too. In advance of the chemo being infused, calm your mind and relax. When the line is attached and the chemo starts to flow down the line into your body, visualise it seeking out the cancer and immediately attacking it. See the chemo as powerful and deadly to the cancer cells. See the cancer melting away as the chemo reaches it.

this approach makes me enthusiastic about treatments

I do this with my eyes open as I am a good day-dreamer and not easily distracted from my imagery by things going on around me. Whether you have your eyes open or closed is your choice, though you will unavoidably be interrupted at times. Depending on the régime, there is usually a lengthy period during which the various agents are infused so there is ample time to imagine the overwhelming of the weak cancer cells.

This approach not only gives me more confidence in the efficacy of the chemotherapy, it also makes me more positive, even enthusiastic about treatments — far better than the dread that often otherwise happens.

Attacking the cancer to reduce its mass or stop its progress

This is a similar method to the one described above, only it is used outside of treatment times. I often used it when I was in a hospital bed or at home. It is a popular approach globally and appears in many CAM programmes. Simply create your relaxed state, then visualise the cancer cells being attacked and either absorbed and dissipated, or otherwise destroyed by some power or force of your choice.

I have enlisted an army of miniature white knights to gallop around in me spearing the cancer

What you imagine as your body's army is up to you. I have employed a number of different armies, including Pacmen (from the old video game) gobbling up the cancer cells. I have enlisted an army of miniature white knights to gallop around in me spearing the cancer, with the cells withering away on the end of their spears. And I have employed a white or blue light, acting like a 'sea of good' seeking out and destroying the clearly bad cancer cells.

The force you choose represents your strong, powerful and highly effective immune cells. Add your emotions into your imagery — be excited as your champions destroy the cancer cells, be proud of your army; see it as strong and unbeatable. The good guys *always* win.

Visualisation guided by another person

Many cancer support organisations convene guided imagery sessions generally similar to what I outline above. The facilitator will use verbal suggestion to help you attain a peaceful state, then will talk you through a visualisation journey, for relaxation or cancer-suppression. It will likely take from 20 minutes to an hour before you return safely and restfully to the room.

Visualisation guided by an audio facility (tape/CD)

Today there are numerous off-the-shelf audio products to help you relax and visualise healing cancer through guided imagery. You can use these alongside self-administered visualisation; they have an advantage over group sessions in that you can do it in privacy and without potential disruption from others. I used various tapes, both to relax and to mentally combat the cancer. You can buy them from many health and book stores.

Guided by a hypnotherapist

Hypnosis is an accepted, useful complementary therapy to help control side-effects of treatments and to help control pain, as well as for imagery to combat the cancer directly. I used it to help programme myself to build my optimism and belief in my ultimate recovery. I went to a hypnotherapist whenever I thought I could benefit from having my imagery and affirmations *reinforced at a deeper level* than I could achieve alone.

Under mild hypnosis, I had the hypnotherapist talk me through a visualisation exercise, or plant and reinforce affirmations over the 60–90 minute sessions. I also had them teach me how to put myself into a mild hypnotic state so I could continue the work alone. I had a session recorded so I could play it to myself at home or in the hospital whenever I wanted. I had just a few sessions then relied on the tape from there on, and on self-guided methods.

many people, notably high-performance athletes, use hypnotherapy to help achieve a wide range of goals

While hypnosis sounds a little other-worldly, in reality it's an easy, relaxing and safe experience. Many people, notably high-performance athletes, use hypnotherapy to help achieve a wide range of goals and objectives.

Be clear with your hypnotherapist about what you want to achieve and why; don't be coy about your condition or your objectives. Hypnotherapists are open-minded. They deal in hope and affirmations. You may choose to write your own affirmations for the hypnotherapist to use on you (as per the suggestions in the next chapter), or ask them to develop something for you.

You'll find directed imagery easy, fun and beneficial. I said in the preceding chapter that I 'kidded myself' into believing in my recovery when the odds were against it. So too did I visualise myself towards recovery.

12

Affirm your future

You may have heard the phrase "If you can *see* it, you can *be* it." It describes the aim and intent of visualisation. Affirmations embody a new phrase: "If you can *say* it, you can *be* it." Affirmations extend the practice of 'minding your language' as introduced in chapter 10, and are an essential companion to visualisation, because it's difficult to visualise positive outcomes when your self-talk is negative. Affirmations work with positive visualisation methods to create a future-affirming point of view.

Affirmations in practice

Affirmations, like visualisation, have been in use a long time. French psychologist Émile Coué (1857–1926) created the most famous and well-known affirmation: "Every day in every way I am getting better and better." He used this and many other affirmations to help hundreds of his patients recover from psychological and physical ailments.

Affirmations are simply short phrases used in a repetitive fashion to help self-programme towards something you want to be (e.g. healthy, wealthy, happy) or to create (e.g. relaxation, success, contentment). They are particularly effective in combatting the psychological cancer, which can otherwise prey on your emotions and sabotage your self-image and hope.

Applying affirmations as a healing tool requires selecting or creating one and repeating it numerous times in a number of sessions. A thousand repetitions is often suggested for a session, but I have had sessions where I probably repeated a selected affirmation 10,000 times or more! That sounds like a lot, but the phrases are very short and the more times you repeat them the faster and deeper they will enter your psyche and become your reality.

Think back to a time in your life when you have wanted to change a habit or behaviour. You had to give it constant attention and repeat the new behaviour numerous times to make it stick. You will have encountered this if you gave up smoking or lost weight by adjusting eating or exercise habits. It's the same process and the same requirement with entrenching affirmations into your being — repetition, repetition, repetition!

Affirmations can play in your mind anywhere, any time. You can repeat one while having your shower or bath, while on transport to and from work, while eating your lunch or while running, walking, gardening or while having treatments. My most memorable affirmation occurred one day in the 1980s when I walked the length of Takapuna Beach and back, repeating "I am healed." I was in the midst of a tough patch, medical treatments were not working well and I really needed help to turn the course of the cancer. It *did* turn shortly after that time, and I have always felt that the Takapuna Beach episode was a key factor.

Principles for effective affirmations

There are some basic principles and guidelines for creating effective affirmations. They must be expressed as positive phrases rather than negative. An affirmation such as "I hate my job" would only create more of what you don't want. It would reinforce your sense of despondency. Turning this *negative affirmation* into the positive "I accept my ideal job" sets the universe into action to support the statement. Adhering to six principles will ensure affirmations are most effective:

1. Phrase them using the *first person singular* wherever possible. Use phrases starting *I am* … or *I can* …. You can only control yourself; it's pointless creating affirmations to try to alter another's behaviours.

2. Phrase affirmations in the *present tense* wherever possible — as if they are happening now.

3. Phrase affirmations in the *most positive way possible*. As with the job example above, avoid 'no', 'don't' and 'not', or you stand to reaffirm what you want to change. Consider the effect that someone telling you, "Don't trip over" or, "Don't drop that plate" might have on the outcome. If they had said, "Walk carefully" or, "Hold the plate," plate

and poise would have been spared — the possibility of failure would not have been introduced. Similarly, instead of saying to yourself "Don't stress out" before an unpleasant test or procedure such as the dreaded bone marrow test, you are better to say to yourself "I am going to handle it well."

4. Make affirmations *short, simple* and *clear*. Long, complicated statements are difficult to internalise.

5. *Use as many of your senses as possible.* As you say or write down affirmations, create mental images that richly and accurately create the feel you want. What do you see, feel, hear, smell and taste?

6. Fill your affirmations with *emotion*. Imagine what it will *feel* like to be healthy again, for instance, as you say words affirming your health. Or if you are focusing on creating other positive things, what does it feel like to be (for instance) happy, strong, self-assured? Don't just imagine the scenario as you utter the words, give it life and power by feeling the emotions that go with the positive words and images.

Examples of affirmations you might use

Relaxation/stress control

- I am calm and relaxed

- I am restful

- I feel soothed and calm

- I am peaceful and tranquil

- I am still and composed

- I am settled and cool

Build optimism and belief in recovery

- I am strong

- I am powerful

- I am resilient

- I am well

- I am supremely confident in my recovery

- I'm feeling better and better every day

- I am robust and durable

- I am healed

Add power to medical treatments as they are administered

- The chemo is destroying the cancer

- Chemo kills cancer every time

- The radiotherapy is killing the cancer

- The treatments are healing me

- I feel the rays (radiotherapy) healing me

- I see/feel the chemo healing my body

Attack the cancer to reduce its mass or stop its progress

- My army is strong and invincible

- The cancer cells are destroyed

- I (see/hear/feel/taste/smell) the cancer cells being destroyed

Affirmations and visualisation combined may be the most potent way to achieve the objectives, but just repeating an affirmation to yourself over and over will have dramatic effects, particularly when you attach positive feeling to the words and to the outcome you desire.

Times, places and approaches of use

Most often, affirmations are internalised — repeated silently in your mind. There are three other approaches I like: self-taped, played through headphones; writing them down (like 'lines' at school); and looking into a mirror and repeating them face-to-face.

Recording selected phrases and *going to bed listening to them through headphones* can be effective and convenient. Going to sleep while listening to an affirmation can work a treat because there is no conscious thought or external distraction. They will go straight to your subconscious and in time become part of your internalised thinking. The subconscious tends to accept what it is told, unlike your conscious mind it has no self-censor, but just takes information like a sponge.

I like *writing affirmations down.* Writing them and seeing them in print seems to send the messages deeper. Write the affirmation 100 times, say it in your mind or out loud as you do so, then read it off the page repeatedly, again either out loud or in your mind.

The third approach is to repeat it while *looking directly in a mirror.* Author Louise Hay recommends this approach. She feels looking at yourself in the eye is the most effective way to get results. I used the method and found it effective, though initially it can feel strange looking yourself in the eye and talking to yourself.

To look *ourselves* in the eye and say "I'm okay!" or "I'm great!" or "I'm well!" does take getting used to. But it is extremely powerful. It is cathartic on a number of levels.

Perseverance is required

The success of affirmations is generally linked to the frequency of their use and the length of time over which they are used. Using them often and with feeling ensures they do all they can to support your cause.

People sometimes stop using affirmations; one main reason is that they become uncomfortable. We all hold a bunch of limiting beliefs about ourselves and challenging these with positive statements creates discomfort. Our limiting beliefs such as hurt feelings, anger, guilt and fear have become entrenched, so we resist positive affirmations. Persevere! The outcomes will be worth it.

going to sleep while listening to an affirmation can work a treat

Where negative self-talk is an entrenched part of your personality, it can be a big ask to change language use. Sometimes people who habitually use negative-speak end up putting themselves down *further* while working to adjust their self-talk. For instance, when finding themselves talking or thinking negatively they might say "I should be able to change this. I must be an idiot!" Avoid this self-deprecating and counter-productive response and hang in with the affirmations, imagery and self-talk to help steer you towards the recovery you seek, and the happy and fulfilled life you want for your life beyond cancer.

Part III

Explore and express yourself

13

Create your future

This chapter details a *life path audit* process to review your present life against your self-assessed ideal life in a structured way, and then identify and do what you need to do, to move towards that ideal. The process can establish additional motivation and resolve to face the battle at hand or ahead. I will weave in my own life path audit I did during my last cancer battle in 2003/4 to help illustrate the process and the benefits.

You can help create your future

I am a great believer in setting visions for the future. I 'saw' all my recoveries from cancer ahead of time. At each new diagnosis, relapse or recurrence, I developed a powerful vision of myself *after* the battle had been won. Thereafter, whatever I had to endure to get to that point would be more bearable. I also had a career and life endpoint to use as my beacon to aim for. It was as bright as it was happy and fulfilling. It was something I would, if required, crawl over broken glass to get to. When you have a vision of what you can become and what you really want, like what you see and receive encouragement and support, you immediately set on a path to over-achieve.

when you have a vision of what you can become and what you really want...you immediately set on a path to over-achieve

The more joy, happiness and sense of fulfilment you feel, the better your immune system will function. The key to experiencing these things is to live in accordance with your natural way of being, relating and creating, as Lawrence LeShan terms it. With a little work you can greatly improve the quality of your life and find your own unique way of living. A seven-step life path audit process can enable you to determine and then start to create your ideal life. This, in turn, may help to overcome your cancer diagnosis — the one supports the other. The seven steps are:

1. Develop a clear sense of your unique purpose.

2. Write a life vision statement for yourself.

3. Establish where you are now in relation to your vision of your ideal life.

4. Develop goals to achieve your vision.

5. Build detailed plans to reach each of your goals.

6. Carry out your plan.

7. Review your progress and celebrate your results!

Creating your future

Step 1: Develop a clear sense of your unique purpose.

Powerful questions to help you better understand your purpose are:

What is worth creating? What is important to you? What do you value most in life? Look into the future. See yourself happy, healthy and fulfilled. What is in your life? Who is in your life?

If you won the lottery today, a big one, what would you do? What would you do differently? What would you stop doing? What would you do more of? Who would you spend more time with?

What would your one dream be if you knew you could not fail? No boundaries or restrictions. No fear of failure. What would it be?

What would you do for free? If you chose to do volunteer work, what would it be and who would you do it for?

The answers to these questions will tell you what you really care about so that you can start to get a sense of how you could create an ideal life congruent with your way of being, relating and creating. They may also point to the answer to the biggest question of all — why you are here on this earth. These questions may take some time to digest, consider and answer well. But they are worth devoting time to, particularly as you spend time in a hospital bed or resting up at home. Try to get beyond the day-to-day issues in your review of them. Use your imagination.

During my own most recent life path audit in 2004 I found answering these questions a big test. My personal life was perfect as far as I was concerned, with a happy marriage to my soulmate Gillian, and great family and friends. But I knew that while I enjoyed some aspects of my work immensely, I had long been dissatisfied with life in the corporate arena. As a general manager in a professional services company I thoroughly enjoyed working with people to achieve objectives. I especially loved helping staff grow and develop, but I loathed managerial politics and posturing, and the insincerity and absence of empathy for people that prevailed within my company's management team. I also knew that I was not *creating* like I wanted to. The business world is often far more competitive than it is creative, and this didn't fit with my needs to create and contribute to the world in a meaningful way.

When I looked at what I would change about my life, if there were no impediments or obstacles, I found myself focusing on my work life and how I might establish employment that could just as easily be what I would do on a volunteer basis. *What did I love to do?* I loved to write, for one. I had already written numerous published articles and most of these were on subjects such as establishing work/life balance, being passionate about work and life, being an empathetic manager worthy of your

during my own most recent life path audit in 2004 I found answering these questions a big test

staff, and how to help staff grow and develop as people. I also yearned to be involved in work that might contribute positively to the needs of people searching for meaning in their lives. For about ten years I had dreamed about writing the book you are reading now, but had little time or energy left to write after my long days in the office.

What meant most to me? I had a lifetime of exploring the meaning and purpose of life. Maybe that was tied to my cancer diagnosis as a teenager, but as long as I could remember the deepest question I wanted to answer was *What's the meaning of my life?* Seeing and helping other people discover their life paths really excited me too. When I asked myself the *winning the lottery* question I found myself listing several activities including writing books, to help other people grow and develop, helping people survive cancer, and being totally happy, healthy and fulfilled myself. I had no idea at this point what job would allow me to pursue my ideal life while still earning enough money to help keep a roof over our heads. As I lay in my bed in the oncology ward or was convalescing at home, I kept writing down any thoughts I had about the subject and let my mind turn them over.

Write down the thoughts that come to you. Keep writing them down as they come to mind until you have a stronger sense of the life you would love to create. Throughout the life path audit you are seeking to establish a sense of *your own* ideal life, which may differ to some extent or even to a great extent from the life you've lived to this point. You'll already start to see that it's a life worth reaching out for and fighting for with everything you have!

Step 2: Write a life vision statement for yourself

The power of a motivating vision statement is that when used in conjunction with goals and actions, it enables you to create almost anything you want. Having considered the questions provided in step 1, carefully write a short phrase that encapsulates the things you've come to understand about what you would be aiming for in your ideal life. If you resolve that you're already living your ideal life, great! Skip now to Chapter 14. If not, read on.

it's your vision so make it perfectly fit you

It's the big picture you're capturing rather than the detail, which will come later. It's *your* vision so make it perfectly fit *you*. When you read it back to yourself you will feel inspired and passionate about the thought and the feel of it. I will give you some examples of life vision statements that might be relevant to other people:

- To help other people achieve their goals (maybe this person could become a life, business and career coach.)

- Be the happiest person in the world (from someone who most values being in a happy state — they will also need to resolve what makes them most happy.)

- To become a renowned painter. (Maybe Picasso had this statement on his mantelpiece?)

- To create world-class gardens. (An avid gardener who loves to create through nurturing and cultivating in the world of plants could spend their life achieving this vision.)

- To care for, protect and nurture animals. (These people will likely be found at SPCAs worldwide, or in veterinary clinics, but they could just as easily be found doing volunteer work for the benefit of animals anywhere.)

- To lead my community. (As cynical as we are about politicians, we need great leaders at local and international levels.)

- To solve the question of the creation of life. (Solving the puzzle of the 'big bang' is well beyond me but someone needs to do it.)

- To be a drummer and a high profile figure in the entertainment world. (Ringo, the Beatles' drummer, once said that if he hadn't ended up in the world's best ever band he might have been found playing "behind the strippers." Drumming wasn't just his job, it was his passion and life.)

These are examples of what vision statements can look like. They may or may not resonate with you. You will have unique needs and values. Your vision statement will reflect what is most important in life to *you*, not to someone else.

At this stage of my life audit process, I decided that all of the needs I had identified for myself were aligned to one theme: helping other people find their way in life and in doing so, helping them and myself become happier and more fulfilled. On reflection this is what had always stirred my passions the most. I therefore compiled a personal life vision for myself as follows:

Phil's Life Vision: *To show people how to live happier and more fulfilling lives.*

Step 3: Establish where you are now in relation to your vision of your ideal life

Be prepared for the possibility of being surprised by what you discover about yourself in establishing your sense of purpose and your life vision statement. The reality for many people is they have long been on a life path that they stumbled upon by accident, by family or peer pressure or by life's circumstances. You may find when you look at your ideal life that you went down a road you would have avoided if you had taken stock earlier. Examples of this are the lawyer who discovers their values don't fit in the confrontational environment they have ended up in, or the accountant who dearly wanted to teach.

As Confucius said, "A journey of a thousand miles begins with a single step." Break down your journey ahead and address each part. If you determine during Step 3 that you are a long way from what you feel is your ideal life, that's okay. It means that you have an exciting road of discovery ahead of you, on which you will find something that will stir your passions, that is worth working towards. Often, though, we are closer to our ideal life than we realise.

moving from a current position to a dream future lifestyle will mean planning well and taking a series of steps towards the vision

To illustrate, consider the accountant who resolves they would love to teach. It may appear initially as though they are at the opposite end of the career spectrum to their ideal, but there may be many overlaps and many ways to transfer their current skills into a teaching profession. Maybe they could find a job teaching part-time at the local college while continuing with their day job for the time being? Maybe they could do *pro bono* teaching at night school to get the experience of teaching? Maybe they could volunteer to teach the helpers at a budget advice service or other community organisation? More often than not, moving from a current position to a dream future lifestyle will mean planning well and taking a series of steps towards the vision. The road may be shorter or longer than we imagine, but the maxim 'it's the journey that counts most' applies here.

In my case as for most people, I was not in a position financially to simply leave my job and start helping people in some still unresolved way to find their ideal life paths. Whatever I did had to have an element of paid work to supplement areas I might be doing for free for a time. At this stage, I started to focus on finding or creating a job that I could move into from my corporate role and would enable me to use my existing skills and experience.

During my research, largely carried out on the internet between hospital stays, I discovered the profession of life, business and career coaching. The closer I looked at it, the more I felt this was a perfect match with my needs and objectives at this time. My research showed that coaches worked with people to help identify life and career visions. They help to achieve goals by removing obstacles and overcoming inertia along the way. I felt I had an ideal background to excel in this area, because I had:

- a lifetime interest in personal and professional development behind me.

- 26 years experience (at that point) facing cancer diagnoses personally and so had addressed issues such as life meaning and my mortality more than most people ever would.

- already coached cancer patients internationally over ten years via internet cancer support sites to help support their recoveries.

- worked in a coaching capacity within leadership roles for most of my career.

- almost 30 years business and management experience to draw on.

- post-graduate business degrees and had carried out several research dissertations on issues such as work/life balance, family-friendly work practices and work satisfaction.

- numerous articles to my name in respected business publications on the kind of issues many coaching clients want to work on.

It became clear that a career in life, business and career coaching would fit my needs and abilities perfectly. However, there were other things I also wanted and needed to achieve in my life. Goals would first need to address surviving the current cancer battle in the first instance, and then the other needs that I would establish.

Step 4: Develop goals to achieve your vision

Establishing some goals is the first key step to realising your vision. You need to write down the key goals that will lead to reaching your vision of an ideal life over time. While visions work from the future back to the present, plans and goals start from your current position and work incrementally from the present into the future. Goals and plans draw from your intellect, whereas your vision comes straight from your heart and is limited only by your imagination.

Goals should always be created and written to be SMART, an acronym for: Specific (have their expected outcomes stated as simply, concisely and explicitly as possible); Measurable (can be assessed to have been successfully achieved or otherwise); Achievable (have outcomes that are realistic given your current situation, resources and time available); Relevant (help you towards your vision which will reflect your desires and aspirations) and Time-bound (which include realistic timeframes within clear achieved-by dates).

Your goals will use the creative tension between your current position and your future vision to pull you towards your future. I suggest you set between six and eight goals to work towards, knowing that when each is achieved you are a big step closer to your vision. Your goals must be relevant to the achievement of your vision and need to be written down. For examples of goals that you might set for yourself, the following are those I developed in support of my new vision statement:

Phil's goals 2004

a) to live a healthy and balanced life

- To survive the cancer diagnosis first and foremost

- To feel a sense of balance between my work and leisure activities which had been absent so often before

b) to be active and creative in generating my success

- Finding my own way of creating was important to me, to enhance my enjoyment of life and to develop a stronger immune system

- With my strong need to achieve I also had to ensure I remained stimulated and had a busy and challenging forward set of activities and goals to reach for

c) to be happy and fulfilled realising my life vision

- Personal happiness and fulfilment were very important to me

d) to be passionate and confident about what I do at all times

- I wanted to ensure that from now on I would only do what made me passionate in life — no more settling for any less!

- Self-belief was also an extremely important thing to ensure I maintained and further developed. I knew that doing what I loved to do would also allow me to feel even more consistently confident in myself and my abilities

e) to help others get passionate and confident about what they do

- I would achieve this through my coaching activities, writing, speaking engagements and any other services I would provide in the company I would form

f) to become a published author of books reflecting my life vision

- You are currently reading the first fruit of this goal; I'm already planning and preparing further books which will reflect my life vision to empower and help inspire people wanting to create more happiness and fulfilment in their lives

g) to become a sought-after coach and adviser

- I would need to establish how to set up business as a coach and to ensure I was the best I could be at delivering coaching services

h) to retain our home and lifestyle while achieving these goals

- This was my 'security' goal, to weigh against all my other goals and ensure we didn't hit Skid Row while I went in pursuit of my goals and life vision

My eight goals incorporated all the things I had resolved I needed, based on the person I was and my values. They included a lot of creativity and a focus on personal happiness and fulfilment, while helping others achieve the same. I also addressed my need for security with my final goal. I knew it was important to allow my head to be in the clouds while keeping my feet firmly on the ground, but I was not prepared to settle for anything less than my dream life from here on.

If you get stuck with the development of your goals, perhaps ask a trusted friend to assist getting them out of your head and into written form, or engage a good life coach.

Step 5: Build detailed plans to reach each of your goals

This is where your goals are made into bite-sized, readily achievable actions. Organised plans of action are the key to all success. *Failing to plan is planning to fail.* Take each goal and write down every step needed to reach it. Put all the plans for the goals together in a format that you can implement each day. Then prioritise the plans. What needs to be done first? What needs to be done today, tomorrow? What can wait but needs other actions to precede it? Write action lists for the week and decide what you want to do today towards the week's action plan. Write down timeframes.

My action list for my Goal 1: 'To live a healthy and balanced life' looked something like this as at 2004:

1. Eat a balanced diet and re-build my weight to an optimum level

2. Continue to develop my life path audit and carry the action plans through (re-aligning my life path was a *need* at this point, not a want)

3. Continue to work with my medical team to make my recovery a reality

4. Take opportunities to rest and relax, and relieve my mind and body from the stresses of the treatments.

On a weekly and daily basis I had sub-actions that I wrote down and carried out. For instance, in terms of action step 1: I weighed myself twice daily, continued to up my calories with advice from the hospital nutritionist, and ensured I took my anti-nausea medication.

In deciding what you need to do, get tough: some of the actions established will have a major impact on your goal, others will have only a small part to play. You might tend to avoid and delay actions you feel awkward about taking, but sometimes these can be the most relevant, so be brave and face them. If you focus only on the trivial matters that are fun, you stand to fail to reach that particular goal. This might dishearten you about achieving your vision. Tips to help you overcome your fears or procrastination include:

- Change the mental picture you have of the necessary action into something fun and exciting, rather than fearful or uncomfortable.

- Imagine the disappointment of *not* achieving your goals and vision — use that to push you to the required action.

- Really imagine the pleasure of reaching your goals and vision. Use the feelings of unbridled joy, happiness and excitement to pull you into action on the steps towards them. Use those senses as described in the visualisation chapter.

- Feel the fear and do it anyway! — the title of my all-time favourite self-help book by Susan Jeffers — herself a cancer survivor. See her words of inspiration within my book, in chapter 18.

Step 6: Carry out your plan

As I said at the outset of this book, it is never enough to know about what you want to do; you must do it. Taking action is at the heart of all success stories in life, and how our dreams and desires become our reality. Having a well constructed plan to create an ideal life is of little value unless it's acted upon with persistence, vigilance and resilience. So on a daily basis, take action towards the goals and enjoy the process!

Step 7: Review your progress and celebrate your results

Circumstances can change and you might get sidetracked from your life audit process at times. You can become off-course for any number of reasons, not the least being elements of the cancer treatment and convalescence.

It's important with any plan of action that you take time regularly to assess how things are going, what actions are being achieved and which are not, and where you are in relation to achieving your goals.

It's simply a case of gently going back to the goals you have established and deciding whether you are getting closer to them. Where you are slipping, think about how you can get back on track. Where circumstances change and new plans are called for, develop these. But be easy on yourself at this time of your life. You won't fail, and things will happen as they should, at the right time — providing you persevere.

Reward yourself along the way as you carry out your plans, achieve your goals and move closer to the vision of your ideal life. Progressive self-rewarding is a great way to motivate you towards achievement. As you reach your goals by self-imposed deadlines, treat yourself to something. Plan ahead what your treat will be and make it something to look forward to. It doesn't need to cost money — it could be taking time out to read a long awaited book, or finally watch films you've recorded ages ago.

Share your achievements. Involve your family or friends in reward outings wherever possible. Encourage them to share in and celebrate your successes with you. In that way they will be active supporters of your pursuit of an altered life path as well as in your recovery from cancer.

Postscript: Some results from my life path audit as at 2006

- I recovered fully from my 2003/2004 cancer battle and regained all the weight, energy and verve I had lost.

- I left my corporate job almost immediately on my return to work in 2005 and began a transition programme to become a life, business and career coach, writer and motivational speaker.

- I travelled to Australia and undertook training as a coach to put a formal structure to all the coaching I had done in various environments, with CoachU (the training arm of CoachInc.com), the world pioneers of coach training.

- I established my company Life Paths Ltd based in Wellington, New Zealand.

- I am currently working with a range of coaching clients on all sorts of coaching issues. At the heart of most of my clients' issues though is the life path one — where are they in relation to where they want to be? This is the common, universal problem to resolve for everyone who wants to live their life to the full.

- I have greatly enjoyed presenting to diverse groups of people to help inspire them to make the most of their lives.

- I am now being, relating and creating in my own unique way. As a result, I am happy and fulfilled like never before in my life. Each day is a new adventure as I live my life on my terms. It will only get better.

- I have enjoyed many celebrations to acknowledge achievements in pursuit of my ideal life and my vision statement so far. Most recently, Gillian and I travelled to the Pacific to relax and reflect for three weeks on the life that was unfolding for us both. I actually took an early draft of this book with me and carried out an edit alongside our hotel pool — with a cocktail in hand! Now that's what I call integrating life and 'work' as God intended!"

To stay focused on your new life path, return to your vision statement often. Put it up on your wall at home, at work or by your hospital bed. Have it in front of you as ongoing inspiration. Sense the happy and fulfilled feelings that achieving your vision and your goals will bring.

The poet WH Auden defined cancer as 'a foiled creative fire.' Reignite your fire during your cancer battle and discover how much you enjoy the experience. Imagine again how wonderful your life will be, every day, when you have created a future ideal life to pursue and love.

14

Humour heals

"A merry heart does like good medicine, but a downcast spirit dries up the bones." Proverbs 17.22

"Let the surgeon take care to regulate the whole regimen of the patient's life for joy and happiness, allowing his relatives and special friends to cheer him, and by having someone tell him jokes." Henri de Mondeville, French surgeon, 1260–1320.

"Always laugh when you can. It is cheap medicine." Lord Byron, poet, 1788–1824.

You no doubt enjoy a good laugh, but do you realise laughter can be an effective coping mechanism and a potent anti-cancer tool? People have long believed in laughter's medicinal properties in disease prevention and cure but little scientific attention was given to it before Norman Cousins released his best-selling book *Anatomy of an Illness* (1979).

Cousins' story is now part of the folklore of mind-body-spirit medicine. An American writer, editor and visionary, Cousins used laughter to help overcome a connective tissue disease called ankylosing spondylitis. He was diagnosed in 1964 with a case so severe that he was given a one-in-five-hundred chance of recovery and a few months to live.

Having read endocrinologist and stress researcher Hans Selye's accounts of how stress harmed health, Cousins decided the reverse must also be true. He resolved to use laughter as a therapy in conjunction with large doses of vitamin C, optimism and the unconditional moral support of his physician. Laughter helped him overcome the excruciating pain of the disease (ten minutes of boisterous laughter alleviated it so that he got two hours of sleep) and ultimately to achieve a complete recovery. His method was to induce laughter frequently by watching the Marx Brothers and episodes of *Candid Camera,* and by having his home-care nurse read him humorous stories.

Cousins used laughter to help heal a depressed immune system as well as a depressed mood, and credited laughter as the prescription that gave him back his life: "(It) is an antidote to apprehension and panic… It creates a mood in which other positive emotions can be put to work too."

As often happens, Cousins received public enthusiasm and acclaim but professional criticism and ridicule from the medical fraternity until 1989, when his views were vindicated by Swedish researcher Lars Ljungdahl, who wrote an article in the *Journal of the American Medical Association*, 'Laugh if This is a Joke.' Ljungdahl concluded "…that a humour therapy programme can increase the quality of life for patients with chronic problems and that laughter has an immediate symptom-relieving effect for these patients, an effect that is potentiated when laughter is induced regularly over a period."

In the years since, evidence from researchers worldwide has shown numerous physiological and psychological benefits of laughter. Muscles in the chest, abdomen, shoulders, neck, face and scalp get a beneficial workout and other parts of the body become more relaxed. This is valuable for patients during the sedentary experience a cancer battle can be, due to fatigue or temporary incapacitation.

laughter enables us to alleviate stress, tension, anxiety, anger and even grief

Laughter enables us to alleviate stress, tension, anxiety, anger and even grief. Like crying, it releases pent-up emotions and can modify our moods: "We don't laugh because we're happy, we are happy because we laugh," philosopher and psychologist William James observed.

It increases immune system function and reduces levels of stress hormones. Studies have found an increase in the amount of natural killer cells (cells that kill cancer cells) in the immune systems of people watching humorous videos.

It is now common to find 'humour therapy' used as an adjunct to other treatments, particularly with cancer patients. In Los Angeles, a 'humour wagon' makes weekly visits to hospitals to entertain children with cancer. The Hospital Satellite Network of Los Angeles has created a television service specialising in humour for hospitals. Called 'Patient America' the programme beams classic comedies and other entertaining features to recovery rooms.

"Men will confess to treason, murder, arson, false teeth or a wig. How many of them will own up to a lack of humour?" Frank More Colby

When I read *Anatomy of an Illness* amidst my cancer battle in the late 1980s, I immediately embraced laughter as an anti-cancer tool and started to build my own humour library. I taped my favourite TV comedies to watch at regular intervals, including re-runs of *MASH, Cheers, Get Smart, Fawlty Towers* and *Monty Python*. Creating situations where I could have a hearty laugh enabled me to keep my spirits up and helped me remain positive and optimistic in the face of some real knockbacks over an 18-month period, including two relapses and a (supposedly) poor prognosis.

laughter helped me establish some control over my situation

Laughter helped me establish some control over my situation. I knew I could consciously elevate my frame of mind — manipulate my point of view for the better — after a time where my moods, emotions and concerns about my predicament had started to rule me.

I could use humour to my benefit by seeing the funny side of everyday events and occurrences while undergoing my treatments and tests. My sense of humour had taken a pounding but resolving to consciously take aspects of the challenge more lightly resulted in my laughing in sometimes unlikely situations, which helped me cope. Four recollections come to mind where I took this approach:

- Before operations under general anaesthetic you have to remove your clothes and don ridiculous paper garments (hat, underpants and shoes) that the hospital provides (for its own comic relief, I have always felt!). You can't help but feel self-conscious and embarrassed wearing those things, but I decided to have a good laugh at my own expense and found my mood lifted. It served to calm my nerves and put me in a frame of mind to better cope with the after-effects of anaesthetic and my recovery from the operation.

"Laugh at yourself first, before anyone else can!" Elsa Maxwell

- When you enter the operating theatre, you suddenly find a whole lot of masked people in green-and-white surgical uniforms, which can be unsettling to say the least. As you look around there is a table full of instruments to be used on you. Your imagination can send your concerns into orbit if you give what you see too much thought. I decided to see those in the room as looking kind of ridiculous, as they do, rather than ghoulish, and this — plus the knowledge that I too looked ridiculous in my paper underwear eased nerves and concerns to the point where I felt positively cheerful before my surgeries, at least until the anaesthetic knocked me out cold.

"Laughter is a tranquilliser with no side-effects" Arnold Glasgow

- Before having a radiculogram test on one occasion (a small needle inserted into the back under local anaesthetic), I was sitting outside the room with my oncology doctor, who was there to observe, waiting for the previous patient to finish. Suddenly from the room came some of the loudest, most hair-raising screaming you ever heard. I had never had this procedure and others in the ward had claimed it was very unpleasant, so naturally my initial thoughts were along the lines of "Oh hell, what am I in for here?" Instead of vocalising my thoughts I turned to my doctor and said "That's nothing, wait until I get in there!" She laughed, but her apprehensive expression told me she wasn't sure if I was joking or not. Her discomfort at the prospect of my response to the procedure allowed me to lighten up greatly and when the screamer exited on a hospital bed, sobbing, I was relatively calm as I went in. As it turned out, the procedure was totally painless anyway, but I'm sure my high spirits helped me take it in my stride.

"Laughter is the sun that drives winter from the human face" Victor Hugo

- Finally, I had been on intravenous fluids in the hospital ward for some days because I had been dehydrated. I was taken away from the oncology ward to have another procedure, and found myself in need of a pee. They were measuring all my liquid outputs so I couldn't simply use the toilet, and had to use a hospital bottle instead. I was handed one and shown to a space surrounded by a material screen like a shower curtain. I must really have had a lot of built-up fluids because I filled the 1-litre bottle in short order. What to do now? I called out to my doctor for another one through the screen, and with gritted teeth, crossed legs and clenched buttocks was handed this.

Then lo and behold, I filled this one and still hadn't finished! I would normally have been embarrassed and self-conscious, but laughing at the situation instead, as I asked for a third bottle from my doctor, sitting as she was in the crowded public waiting area, allowed me to relax, physical discomfort notwithstanding. My doctor couldn't believe I needed a third bottle but provided it anyway. By the time I got to the procedure I had laughed myself into a jovial mood and it was another stress-free and pain-free experience.

"Laughter is the most healthful exertion" Christoph Wilhelm Hufeland

I can recall many experiences during my cancer battles when I was able to turn potential embarrassment, discomfort, fear, depression or trepidation into relaxed and jovial situations where I felt in control of and comfortable with my situation by using humour and laughter. Simply changing the way I responded to these common hospital experiences had a dramatic impact on my mood and ability to cope. I never forgot I was in a fight for my life and I remained clear, focused and motivated in my quest to beat the disease, but in making light of these sorts of experiences I was unconsciously diminishing the cancer itself in my mind, which took power away from it. This helped me to concentrate on positive outcomes, rather than on concerns about how or if I would achieve my recovery.

"He who laughs, lasts" Mary Pettibone Poole

Several studies have shown that young children laugh up to 400 times a day, while adults typically laugh only 15 — 20 times per day. We somehow lose our inclination to laugh as we grow older, often along with our spark and passion for life — a real pity. A cancer diagnosis will test your sense of humour further without question, so deciding to employ laughter to elevate your mood and return humour to your life will be very beneficial.

Building your own laughter library is a simple and useful thing to do to ensure that you have access to funny material when you want it. Humour is something that is totally personal — what makes me laugh might not do the same for you and vice versa. These days there is a wealth of humorous CDs, DVDs, videotapes, books and magazines in shops and on the internet, or for borrowing from your local library, friends and family, or your cancer support organisation.

I urge you to start your own humour library, filling it with comedy TV and radio shows and movies that you have most enjoyed throughout your life. Many of the classic shows from yesteryear have been re-produced and are available now. Most cancer wards have their own TV/DVD/videotape facilities and also humorous shows on tape. Check out their collection and enjoy those that appeal to you as often as you can. As you work on the serious business of beating cancer, try to see the funny side of daily life as well.

15

Write for release

"The act of putting pen to paper encourages pause for thought, this in turn makes us think more deeply about life, which helps us regain our equilibrium." Norbet Platt, author.

Creative activities can be great respites from a cancer battle, and are stimuli for our natural healing processes. Many cancer patients participate in one or more creative pastimes such as music, art, dance, sculpting, pottery, acting, gardening and writing to those ends, or simply for the pleasure of it. Two of the most popular pursuits with cancer patients are expressive writing, the subject of this chapter, and music, the subject of the next. They are accessible, engage people completely and allow their deepest thoughts, feelings and concerns to be explored.

Psychoneuroimmunology research has shown direct health benefits to result from expressing life experiences in writing. James W Pennebaker is professor of psychology at the University of Texas and a foremost researcher on the effect of writing on health. In 1986, he found college students who wrote about emotional experiences had fewer doctors' visits and less illness throughout the following year. Doctors Roger Booth and Keith Petrie, at the University of Auckland, have found writing to provide greater immune responsiveness, linking writing about personal traumatic events with a stronger antibody response to the Hepatitis B vaccine.

Dr Pennebaker: "Standing back and exploring your thoughts and feelings about your major life experiences can have profound effects on your physical and mental health. An impressive body of research finds that when people write about traumas, negative or positive turning points in their lives, or simply write about their life stories, they derive great benefits."

These are more than an emotional outlet and respite from stress. Writing can encourage learning; insights and understanding which helps us put our life's events into perspective.

I once participated in a writing workshop, conducted through the Cancer Society of New Zealand. The workshop *Your life… Your story* provided a forum to write about aspects of our cancer experiences and to share them with the group. The workshop functioned as much as a support group as a creative outlet.

writing can encourage learning; insights and understanding which helps us put our life's events into perspective

Everyone's experiences provided the others with insights about cancer's impacts and with new ideas on coping. If you can find — or start — one, a writing workshop can be a good way to begin to incorporate writing as part of your cancer recovery programme.

But there are numerous ways expressive writing can be approached without attending a workshop. Some people write poetry about their feelings or experiences, others write songs or keep diaries of events impacting on them and on others battling cancer alongside them. Here are three writing approaches I have gained much satisfaction from.

First approach: narrative to explore, express and release negative emotions

Being diagnosed with cancer can be isolating and lonely. This changes if you share a hospital room with other patients, as you become privy to what they are going through, including their diagnosis and prognosis updates from doctors, and their intimate times with families and friends.

You quickly come to realise that you are one of many with the same fears, trepidations, shock and grief at this time and that in some ways your experience is a collective one. This gives some comfort but at the same time, more emotional distress. It is almost impossible not to be touched by the unfolding stories of those around you.

Your feelings about your own predicament, as well as others', can be explored with the first approach to writing. Writing about your daily experiences and how you feel about them provides a measure of understanding, release and healing. Transposing what you experience and feel into written form is achieved by adopting a phrase of your choice as a prompt, then just writing.

Here are five examples of prompts with an illustrative piece that I wrote:

- "I am scared. What scares me most about my current situation is…"

- "I was deeply concerned by my latest test results…"

- "I was angered by a doctor's comments to me today…"

- "Today I witnessed a touching scene…"

- "What affected me most today was…"

September 12

What touched me most today was…

I spoke to Mrs Betty Jones [not real names] in the ward's tea room. Though in her 70s and quite thin and drawn, she has a cheerful, alert and kindly disposition and has been terrific support to her cancer patient husband Bill who has been in the bed across from me all week. Bill, who moves in a slow, stooped shuffle, has been confused and disoriented since arriving. Betty shared with me that Bill was admitted with a melanoma but the disease had spread through his body. Sadly, he is terminal and probably only has weeks to live, but neither Betty nor her granddaughter Angela (a 20 year old who has worked in tandem with Betty all week, sitting beside Bill) has told him this. Betty said they don't want to add to his worries until and unless absolutely necessary. I noticed a band aid on Betty's arm, the type you get after a blood test, so I questioned her about it. She told me she has recently been diagnosed with cancer herself, and that hers too is terminal. She has not told Bill either. She said she wants to focus on Bill for now and on allowing him to live as good a life as possible.

The selflessness of this and the closeness of their relationship moved me deeply. I gauged from their conversations that they have spent a lifetime of sharing, giving to each other and growing together, and now that both their lives are in the twilight stage she has put aside her own fears, needs and concerns to make his final days as normal and comfortable as possible. That's real love and partnership. I thought too of Angela, who held Bill's hand whenever Betty was out of the room, and what strength and understanding she must possess to know of the plight of her loved grandparents yet still choosing to be there, smiling with them, with her quiet, caring presence. I returned to my bed and pulled the curtains. I cried quietly so the Joneses couldn't hear me from across the room.

Second approach: narrative describing good results, outcomes and progress, to amplify positive emotions

Expression of both positive and negative emotions has been shown to stimulate our immune systems and to contribute to feelings of equilibrium and wellness. It's therefore beneficial to frequently acknowledge, express and reinforce the experiences that stimulate our *positive* emotions.

This second example uses a narrative to express and reinforce positive emotions, taken from the time that I discovered I could be harvested for stem cells. I take the liberty of extrapolating the already positive results I had received to symbolise my power over the disease and the inevitability of success in achieving my remission.

> October 10
>
> Great news this week! Firstly, my blood results came in and I am able to be harvested for stem cells. My medical team had been down-beat about the chances of my blood counts reaching the level required to enable a harvest. After all, the counts were at zero just a couple of days before. As the harvest process took place, with my blood being extracted and my stem cells filtered into bags, the nurse reminded me that there was no guarantee the stem cells within the extract would be sufficient to enable a transplant. I had received so much chemotherapy over the years that I was not a good prospect, she said. Despite others' scepticism I felt confident about the process working out for me.
>
> The next day I was visited by a very excited specialist calling me a star. My harvest was not only successful and adequate in volume; she said it was the highest harvest they've ever had in the hospital! I have enough stem cells for a number of transplants. This was pleasing but not surprising to me. I had told them earlier not to worry; that I would do my bit as long as they did theirs. And now we can start the high dose chemotherapy in the full knowledge that it will do its job perfectly, with the subsequent stem cell transplant ensuring my body recovers from the process. I'm pumped because this shows the medical team I mean business, that when I say I will recover fully I mean it. My recovery and cure are inevitable. I rule!!! Onwards!

Third approach: expressing gratitude to promote positive expectations and emotions

In coaching we talk about the value of having an 'attitude of gratitude,' which simply means taking time to count our blessings rather than focusing on our life's trials and tribulations. This is useful at any point in our lives, but when battling cancer it can help focus our thoughts, feelings and expectations on life-affirming matters that will inherently support the positive outcomes we seek. Each day, take time to reflect on those things that you are grateful for, write them down and acknowledge them.

November 8

[Prompt] Today I reflected on my life and I found myself grateful for:

my loving wife and family who are caring for me through this encounter

my friends and colleagues who visit me and send messages of support

my skilled and inclusive medical team who are helping me beat the disease

the wisdom we have been given to develop the technology that is helping us all in the battle

the genuine concern for my health that I receive from complete strangers in the ward and throughout the hospital

other patients' most intimate experiences and feelings that they share with me every day

my strength of will which is helping me to cope with the hard times and to retain positive expectations for the outcome

my passion for life which makes each day exciting and adventurous

As I discussed earlier, there is no need to try to be perpetually upbeat and thankful for *everything* in your life right now. I would not recommend being grateful for having cancer, for instance! Why would you be? It's an uninvited, unwanted incursion into your life. But reflecting on the genuinely positive things in your life will help you realise that things are not all bad and that you still retain control over a lot and are supported in *all* your endeavours.

"I love writing. I love the swirl and swing of words as they tangle with human emotions." James Michener

These are all examples of approaches to expressive writing I have preferred over others within my cancer recovery programmes. Try these and also others such as poetry or songwriting, and work out what resonates best with you. Whatever expressive writing approach(es) you adopt, six guidelines will help them work best for you:

1. Wherever you write, ensure you are physically comfortable and, if you are concerned at the prospect of becoming emotional in the presence of others, find somewhere private so that you express rather than repress your feelings. When you write about touching encounters, particularly if you are not emotionally open or expressive by nature, writing can become uncomfortable and confronting for you too. Try not to put your writing aside or to resist your emotions if this happens; allow yourself to persist and to express what you feel.

2. There are no hard-and-fast rules about how long to write to derive either pleasure or health benefits. Sometimes you might write for five minutes, at others you might write for an hour or more. On average, people write for twenty to thirty minutes in a session. Before you do write, though, give yourself a little time to reflect on the events of the past day or week.

3. Try to be as detailed as you can about the events you are writing about. Aim to link what occurred with the feelings and emotions that arose from them, rather than just writing the sequence of events. *"He said ..., she cried, he held her ..."* etc, describes only part of the process and omits the element that leads to *feeling* the scenario you have observed.

4. Expressive writing requires no self-editing. Stopping to analyse or critique your writing or to review your spelling, grammar or word structure will stop the flow. The *process* is far more important than the words that flow from this writing.

5. If you find your writing starts to resemble a set of complaints, stop and start again. *"They served me tea today that was cold, the eggs were runny and I was woken five times last night by noisy nurses"* may reflect the facts, but it will do little to ease tensions and access the feelings within you. Narrative that explores one of your complaints further and that taps into your humanity will serve you better:

    > I was woken by noisy nurses five times last night. At first I was angry, but then I realised that they were tending to the needs of Mr Smith across from me who had become very ill. He had a number of relapses and I think came close to the brink. The nurses

who tended to him fought with everything they had to relieve his pain and anguish. I recalled him and his wife sitting holding hands the day before; they have been together for 40 years and are clearly very much in love. It breaks my heart to see this couple being separated by illness. Not everyone finds that kind of love and closeness in their life's relationship. I guess it's all part of the cycle of life, but it seems to me tragic for it to have to end.

6. Finally, date and keep all your writing. Later, when your cancer battle is over and some time has passed, your writings will be a terrific spur to reflection that can contribute to your ongoing psychological healing process.

16

Raising spirits with music

The philosopher Friedrich Nietzsche said that music was one of the arts which sharpened our sense of participation in life, and gave life meaning and purpose. Like so many mind-body-spirit practices, music is at once both pleasure and therapy. Music has moved me in ways that few other things have, and it has helped me greatly to cope with cancer.

There is no culture that lacks music and it has long played an essential part in social interaction. In ancient Greece, music was an important part of life and the Greek analysis of the effect of music went very deep. Greeks considered that the right type of music was a powerful instrument of education which could alter the characters of those who studied it, inclining them towards "inner order and harmony".

> *[music] provides relief from pain and nausea, promotes sleep and appetite, reduces anxiety…and promotes an overall sense of wellbeing*

They also gave music a medical value. They saw it as a way to draw out and release strong emotions, thereby helping people achieve a state of equilibrium and consequently, wellness.

'Medicine for the soul'

Music can play a big part in enriching your daily life, and in supporting your recovery from cancer. It has laughter's ability to make you feel better and has shown many of the same physiological benefits as laughter, and meditation. That is, it provides relief from pain and nausea, promotes sleep and appetite, reduces anxiety, lowers heart rates, breathing and blood pressure, and promotes an overall sense of wellbeing.

Meanwhile, like the creative pursuit of writing discussed in the preceding chapter, music can also open and reveal emotions which are trapped within. Plato said it well: *"Music is a moral law. It gives a soul to the universe, wings to the mind, flight to the imagination, a charm to sadness, gaiety and life to everything."*

I used music as therapy throughout my cancer encounters. Being a music lover, I used it naturally and intuitively to help me release tensions, express emotions, overcome depression and assist with crucial decisions.

Releasing tensions

When I was first diagnosed with cancer I was still a teenager, with more energy than I knew what to do with. Naturally my diagnosis created tensions, concerns and grief that scattered my energies and upset whatever semblance of equilibrium I might have had to that point. I needed a catalyst to help centre me. Fortunately I was already playing the drums in a band, and pounding out the rhythm helped me rid myself of many tensions. I also enjoyed listening and dancing to a lot of live music. It was the late 1970s and New Zealand's music scene was alive with bands. Dancing, playing and listening to music at the time were ways for me to unwind and ground myself.

Emotional expression

Emotional expression was never my strong suit — early on and for a long, long time I was best described as repressed. Though I had strongly-felt emotions to contend with, I kept them locked inside. Like everyone, I needed some way to experience and release them and together with my writing, music greatly helped me fulfil this need. By choosing a style and tone of music that related to what I was feeling, I drew out and expressed emotions. As far as I was concerned it didn't matter if I laughed or cried, because no one could see me. People who express themselves easily and naturally find this difficult to understand, but I know I am not alone in needing an external intervention to enable me to express myself. I have found a lot of my fellow cancer patients tend towards emotional repression — though there are many exceptions, of course.

Overcoming depression

Music has been 'instrumental' at times in taking me out of a depressed state. I was 23 when this was demonstrated to me most vividly. I had moved cities for a new job, from Auckland to Wellington. I knew virtually no one; the weather was gloomy for weeks on end; the lumps under my armpits were larger than ever and the realisation that one day I would be required to face my prognosis also haunted me. I was the most depressed I had ever been.

I decided to play some of my records. I pulled out a bundle of my most cheerful ones and started listening. To my astonishment, my mood went from one of despair and loneliness to one of happiness and elation. I began dancing around the lounge of my flat, my head whirling, my heart pumping as I started to laugh with joy. If the neighbours had seen they might have called the police, concerned that I'd lost my marbles. Temporarily maybe I had, but it felt wonderful.

This experience reinforced for me the power of music to improve my moods in a dramatic way, and too, my ability to control and change my moods and point of view at will. These lessons would serve me particularly well later in the decade when I did become very ill.

Overcoming fear and paralysis in decision-making

As with every cancer patient, I have had to make decisions that would impact the course of my life in a direct way. Should I accept a régime of chemotherapy being recommended by the doctors, in the knowledge that it could damage one or more major organs? Should I undergo a radiotherapy régime that would increase the risk of heart disease downstream? Should I opt for less invasive but unproven measures? Decision-making with potential life-and-death consequences will always be stressful, but using music as a calming, stabilising or resolve-building catalyst really helped, and helped me face the doctors' rounds too.

My approach was to play gentle, relaxing music to help calm me when I needed my decisions to be made in a more considered frame of mind. I played fast and energetic music to pump myself up and put me in 'fight' mode when I felt the need to face impending news with a forward-looking, defiant attitude. If the news was good, it reinforced my heightened spirits. If it was not good, I wasn't devastated because I 'knew' in my defiance I could navigate my way out somehow. I was steeled to cope with the battle and to better position myself for a recovery.

Professional music therapy

My use of music for my recoveries has always been intuitive and loosely structured. There are also structured and facilitated approaches to the use of music as therapy, which have the potential to help cancer patients explore deeper issues. Professional music therapy has developed over several decades to the point where it is now well considered to help restore equilibrium and wellness by international mainstream cancer support.

Music therapists hold to the medicinal value of music as espoused by the ancient Greeks. The New Zealand Society for Music Therapy works with a range of people including cancer patients. Daphne Rickson of the society has written to explain what music therapy is and does:

> Throughout the world, hospitals and cancer clinics have incorporated music therapy in their work with cancer patients. Music therapy gives people with cancer an opportunity to develop creative expression enabling them to mourn, grieve, improve their mood, celebrate life; to cope with and find meaning in their situation. Music is helpful in the management of pain and anxiety since it can touch people deeply, help them relax and therefore heal. Increasingly researchers are discovering scientific evidence, particularly in the biochemical field, to support what music therapists and others believe — that listening to and playing music is also beneficial for the immune system.
>
> While carefully chosen recorded music can be used to achieve some of the goals outlined in the previous paragraph, music therapists usually engage their patients in some kind of musical interaction — examples include listening to and talking about music, playing instruments together, song writing and compiling life story tapes for families. Music therapy programmes that include families can really enhance communication between family members — experiences of past events can be linked to songs that are being played, lives can be reviewed, and people are helped to talk about the things that are important to them. As people become more creative they become more expressive. For those who have strong emotions rendering them unable to speak, songs can provide a channel for reminiscence and expression.
>
> Given the power of music to facilitate positive change, it is not surprising that some researchers argue that music used inappropriately can also aggravate pain. While it is unlikely that listening to favourite music can do harm, it might be helpful for cancer patients to listen to their music collection with 'new' ears and to consider how particular tracks are affecting them. On the other hand, it might be helpful to work with

a music therapist. Music therapists are trained to identify the most appropriate music for a given situation, are highly skilled musicians, and can competently facilitate musical and other forms of communication with patients and their families.

To find out more about music therapy and music therapists, go to the New Zealand Society for Music Therapy website at www.musictherapy. org.nz or contact Daphne Rickson at D.J.Rickson@massey.ac.nz.

Guided imagery and music (GIM)

Another approach to the use of music for cancer patients is to combine it with imagery. A respected facilitated approach to GIM is the Bonny Method of Guided Imagery and Music. Described as a music-assisted mode of self-exploration and therapy, the Bonny Method was conceived and developed by Helen L Bonny, who combined relaxation techniques and classical music selections to elicit responses from patients in the early 1970s at the Maryland Psychiatric Research Center, Baltimore, USA.

The Bonny Method uses sequenced classical music within a one-to-one session conducted by a trained facilitator. After discussing things with you, the facilitator provides relaxation and focusing suggestions to assist you into a relaxed state.

[the method] provides spiritual and emotional insights as well as a sense of healing and wellness

Then you listen to the music and describe the images, sensations, feelings, and awareness it evokes. The facilitator, also listening to the music, helps to focus and support your image experiences in a variety of ways. At the close of the music, the facilitator assists your return from the expanded state of consciousness and through discussion, helps integrate the experiences evoked by the music.

The method provides spiritual and emotional insights as well as a sense of healing and wellness. *Journal of Music Therapy* (USA) reported a study that found that the method was effective in improving the mood and quality of life of cancer patients. Another study, at the University of Rochester Medical Center, found that cancer patients undergoing bone marrow transplants, who experienced music-assisted relaxation and imagery, reported significantly less pain and nausea and their new bone marrow took hold faster, with the average time until patients began producing their own white blood cells being two days earlier than the control group.

My fellow cancer survivor Joanna Booth used music for creating wellness on her own, then employed the Bonny Method of GIM with other creative pursuits in her battle with and recovery from pancreatic cancer. She ultimately trained in and still works with the method. Joanna describes her experiences and the benefits:

> I read Bernie Siegal's books [Love, Medicine & Miracles; Peace, Love & Healing — mind-body-spirit classics] and Bernie recommended music for healing, so Roger [Booth] taped Beethoven's string quartets and Sixth Symphony and the music accompanied me to hospital. I played them every day, all day, and found that each day I had a different emotional response to the music — sometimes to the same music, which, one day would make me feel sunny, and the next would have me weeping uncontrollably. Photos of all our cats completed my 'wellness room' [surely proving Nobel Peace Prize winner Albert Schweitzer's words "There are two means of refuge from the miseries of life: music and cats." author.]

> After hospital, the music continued, and Haydn string quartets were added to the mix. I would fall asleep with the music and awaken as soon as it stopped. Somehow, the music soothed me in innumerable ways, and promoted restful sleep and healing. Classical music has a clear, apprehensible structure, with beginning, middle and end well defined, yet allows and encourages a great deal of emotion to be felt and also worked through as the music progresses.

> Another important stage was to get out into the garden, and I did this after ten days home from hospital. Even though it was difficult and painful there still was that sense of almost exhilaration and then contentment as I got myself thoroughly and happily dirty tending to the plants. These two things, gardening and music, maintain my wellbeing. I cannot live without either. The cats also are important — such a delight to have them around, doing all their catty things.

> Two months on, I found that Helen Bonny was, with three trainee assistants, giving an all-day seminar and workshop on her Guided Imagery and Music at the Auckland University Centre for Continuing Education. After her first sentence, I knew I had come home. GIM sessions, both in a weekly group and one-on-one followed, and much was revealed and worked with. I expanded my sense of self. Training in the Bonny Method of GIM followed, and archetypal experiences during my sessions were the norm, as well as the nuts and bolts of working with life experiences

and changing my whole belief system and attitudes. My world view was challenged repeatedly, and insisted upon expanding and becoming more fluid, more flexible.

As life progresses, I continue to feel that I am coming home to myself; an expanded and more aware sense of self, and as a result of the hard work with GIM and the grace which came with the imagery, the cancer patterns have been transformed into a more nurturing and creative energy. I continue to heal and to expand my world view.

To learn more about the Bonny Method of GIM or where you can access the method in New Zealand, contact Joanna Booth at joanna.booth@xtra. co.nz, ph 09 445 7647.

"Music is the shorthand of emotion" Leo Tolstoy

I saw something that further reinforced for me the power of the use of music. I was in Wellington Hospital's oncology ward receiving chemotherapy and antibiotics, resting at that moment in the dayroom early one evening. Two rough-and-ready Māori guys were talking together in the room with me, one a cancer patient and the other his visitor. I heard the visitor asking "Have you managed to get *it* out yet bro?" "Nah, not yet," he responded. "No worries, bro, no worries, we'll get it out of you."

I wondered what on earth they were talking about. I returned to my cubicle and did a few things to prepare for the evening. Then as I walked back towards the dayroom, I could hear music. A man was singing and strumming a guitar. As I got to one of the other cubicles, I saw the Māori patient laying on his bed, crying his eyes out; his visitor was sitting next to the bed, singing a ballad to him.

The meaning of their earlier conversation dawned on me instantly and I was agape. The memory of that fleeting encounter remains one of the most moving in my years amongst other cancer patients.

Your music will serve you well

The need to open up our emotional channels is major when we have cancer; emotional expression is more important than ever before. It is also a time when we can learn to vent what we have long kept inside us, and to develop greater awareness of ourselves and the way we live our lives and interact with those around us, as alluded to by Daphne Rickson and Joanna Booth. Music is a great stimulus to help with these processes.

Your tastes in music are unique to you; people are as different in their musical preferences as they are in what makes them laugh. You may choose to use music in an unstructured, intuitive way — or to try structured applications of music such as music therapy or GIM. Whatever you decide, why not start to explore what music makes you feel happy, what relaxes you, what energises you and what makes you feel stronger and more in control? What you learn from your exploration will help you to enlist music to your cause, no matter what approach or combination of approaches you select.

If your music collection is small, why not invest in some more to start building a music library to sit alongside your humour library? Use music to cheer yourself up, to escape, to lift you out of depression, to ease and remove stress, to resolve you in your challenges along the way and maybe to help you discover more about yourself, as Joanna Booth, I and many other cancer patients and survivors have done with much success.

Part IV

Life after cancer

17

Post-treatment challenges

The moment arrives; your treatments are complete and you are released from the hospital system. The mix of emotions that arise when this long-dreamed-of day comes can take you by surprise. What was initially a dreaded and feared place often became your safe haven. Despite some painful memories and associations, it is the place where you received nurturing and caring and more individual focus and attention than you may ever have had in your life. As you exit the hospital with a follow-up appointment form in hand, you may be filled with conflicting feelings of elation and apprehension.

The point at which you move from cancer patient to cancer survivor is not definitive. Most people consider themselves cancer survivors when they are in remission, but the doctors will err towards caution even after treatments are completed. The most to expect is to be declared 'in remission,' which means no discernible disease remains. It's sometimes held that after five years in full remission you may be considered cured, but cured is a word you will seldom hear from the mouths of medical professionals.

> *The point at which you move from 'cancer patient' to 'cancer survivor' is not definitive*

If conventional medicines have been exhausted and haven't effected a remission, you have big decisions to make about what you choose to do next. You will need to decide how you wish to live your life, in particular whether your primary focus might be continuing your quest for a full recovery through other means, or the enhancement of the quality of your life, or a combination of the two. There are still treatment options open to you. It may be possible to participate in a clinical trial of a new, as yet unproven anti-cancer product within your hospital or another further afield. There are also a range of unproven alternative treatment offerings that you may identify through research, and pursue.

Life continues, but maybe not as you knew it

All going to plan, though, you will now have been declared to be in remission. Your energies begin to return, your hair starts to grow back (if you lost it), your wounds are healing, disease symptoms and treatment effects are resolving.

Your feelings, however, may not recover as fast as your body. At the beginning of this book, I wrote about the misconceptions people harbour about cancer and what a cancer battle might be like.

many people's feelings don't recover as fast as their bodies

Misconceptions also abound about how you will feel and what you will want to do *after* treatments. Reality is that it's impossible ahead of time to know how you will feel and react. People are adaptable and many cancer survivors do successfully return to life as they knew it, quickly picking up where they left off before their diagnosis, returning to their routines and perfectly content to do so. For others, re-entry into 'normal' life presents challenges.

As you endeavour to re-integrate, deep questions can arise and plague your mind. What did everything that has happened mean in the context of my life? What am I going to do now? Where am I going in my life? What has my life meant and what does it mean that I survived while others didn't? Facing your mortality for an extended period in a place where others were facing theirs can change your outlook on life forever. Haunting memories of treatment régimes, operations and the extreme highs and lows of the cancer experience have a lasting effect too.

Emotional and spiritual disquiet often play on cancer survivors the most, but physical effects also remain. Some residual tiredness and lethargy are common and may continue for months. Memory and concentration can be affected. A colloquial term 'chemo-brain' has been coined for the condition that about a quarter of chemotherapy recipients can experience, involving periodic difficulties in concentrating and collecting thoughts.

And your body's appearance may have altered. An amputation, organ removal or diminished body functioning can be permanent reminders that you have battled for your life. For some, the physical changes will have altered their sense of self and maybe lessened their self-esteem.

Reminders at every turn

Contributing to survival anxieties are the fears that can re-emerge after a cancer battle is completed. Fears usually peak early on, when we are first diagnosed and become anxious for our very lives, for the first time in our lives. During the treatment process, our fears diminish to some extent with the comfort of knowing that action is being taken to address the cancer. After treatments cease, however, with nothing being done now to combat the disease, fears may be re-kindled.

Meanwhile, we fear a recurrence, with any pains or unusual symptoms triggering anguish and concern. Our GP takes a much closer interest in anything that is ailing us too, as we are a known former cancer patient. A simple cold or flu bout can result in blood tests or further investigations 'just in case.' Life insurance becomes impossible to secure other than at exorbitant rates and with cancer-related disclaimers and this in turn can compromise other financial applications. We can be scrutinised closely and sometimes discriminated against at job interviews. All in all we find the label of 'cancer patient' difficult to shed.

a clean bill of health is a relief until you remember you have to repeat the process again in a few months, and in a few months after that

For the first year or two after treatments cease, follow-up checks back at the hospital are frequent, usually 3 or 4-monthly. At each check-up, having been out of the hospital system for some months, you return to it. As well as being intrinsically stressful, the return can stir other feelings. The medical team that nurtured you like a member of its own family now either doesn't recognise you (you have hair again, you have regained weight, and you simply look well), or pay you only a passing attention as they walk by. They are concentrated on the new batch of patients. You appreciate that it's a good thing not being a part of the cancer ward's fold any longer, but at some level you may feel abandoned and a little forlorn.

During these check-ups, no matter how well you feel in yourself, waiting to be seen by the doctors, to receive blood test and x-ray results and your physical examination inevitably brings back memories of your world as a cancer patient. Consciously or unconsciously you harbour concerns that one of the test results will show something irregular. A clean bill of health is a relief until you remember you have to repeat the process again in a few months, and in a few months after that.

Then there are flashback triggers to contend with. Certain noises, smells, sights or tastes can take you back to the hospital, mentally and emotionally. For me, a certain type of orange drink that I used to take oral chemotherapy is now unpalatable. The buzzing noises emitted by some machines can transport me back onto the tables where I received radiotherapy. These sometimes painful and unpleasant memories do fade in time, but 'just forgetting' the whole experience is not a realistic expectation.

The expectations of others

In the meantime, everyone back in the world will expect you to 'return to normal' now that you are restored to health. That means being the 'you' they knew before the cancer battle, behaving the way you did and having the same traits and interests that you did back then. In my experience, that isn't always possible.

For casual friends, acquaintances and workmates, life has gone on much as it was before your cancer encounter. There is no way that they can understand what you have been through, what you have experienced and how these things may have affected and perhaps changed you.

challenges [when] re-adjusting to your work environment often arise

Challenges re-adjusting to your work environment often arise. After an encounter with your mortality, coping with and tolerating people politics and the pettiness that can arise in human interactions can become far more difficult than before, or even untenable as the absolute pointlessness of it becomes clear when weighed against the big issues you have been facing.

When I got back to my place of work once after recovering from a stage 4 cancer battle, I found myself confronted by someone on the warpath for the person who had taken her pen. She was livid, touring the office looking for the culprit. As she finished scanning my desk, storming away to other parts of the office, the realisation that re-integrating would be harder than I thought was more than evident to me.

Relationship conflicts can arise with your spouse, family and closest friends too. They have gone through the cancer battle with you, constantly on call and on edge, acting as your rock when you were incapacitated or weak from the disease or treatments. During the treatment process they were happy to provide you with unconditional support and attention to help you back to recovery. Now that you are considered to be well, they anticipate you will return immediately to your old self. Just wanting you to get on with it, they can struggle to accept that you need more time to adjust and work through the emotional issues stemming from the cancer battle. They may fail entirely to understand your need to take time out to re-evaluate your life.

Their feelings and responses arise in part too because of the grave fears and anxieties they held for you when you were ill. Now that you have recovered, those anxieties, buried to date for fear of affecting your recovery, need venting. While this is a perfectly understandable part of *their* recovery process, it can be at odds with your need to take stock and to find your own way forward. As a result of these conflicting needs, serious communication breakdowns can occur — creating friction, guilt and disharmony on both sides, with temporary or permanent relationship consequences.

Overcoming survivorship woes

The many challenges of 'surviving cancer survival' outlined above have had relatively little research attention internationally. Sydney University's Centre for Values, Ethics and the Law of Medicine is one institution that has undertaken useful research, with interesting and perhaps predictable findings. Emeritus Professor of Surgery Professor Miles Little, who has led this research since 1996, considers a quarter to a third of all cancer survivors may find that the troublesome aspects of cancer and its survival affect the quality of their lives in significant ways:

> …for some survivors at least, survival can be a downward spiral. Survivors feel different — different to the way they were before the cancer, and different to others who haven't had cancer. Confronting the reality of death makes them view life and other people in new ways. They may not have the same interest and commitment to the things that seemed important before cancer. They may therefore not perform as they used to, whether working in a job, being a lover, running a household, looking after a family or playing sport. When people don't perform well, they may lose the respect of others, and then tend to perform even less well. And so the cycle goes, toward an increasing loss of self-respect, and a decreasing willingness to take on challenges, and eventually toward inertia and what seems like depression.

161

Too many cancer survivors exit the hospital system unprepared for life after cancer and unaware of the issues they may be about to face. Hospital systems rarely involve themselves in the patient's life once they have achieved their objectives to restore physical health. But cancer survivorship can present real challenges.

Given the range of issues that can arise it is not surprising to find some degree of 'survivorship depression' and disorientation after treatments cease. It is normal, relatively common and understandable given that in some respects our very sense of identity, of ourselves and the world we live in has changed. It can be very disconcerting to realise that you no longer fit with or relate to aspects of your former life. Despondency and depression can easily lead to feelings of helplessness and hopelessness and a further compromised immune system, if some semblance of order is not regained.

The solution lies in the same approach for successfully coping with the cancer battle itself: attitude and action. The benefits of the perspectives and mind-body-spirit measures presented in this book go well beyond coping with and fighting cancer. They are life-affirming, quality-of-life enhancing catalysts of the highest order.

Adopting the following attitudes and taking the following actions, all of which will now be familiar to you, will help you navigate your way through the transition and reintegration process.

Attitudes

Affirm and accept that:

- You can and will cope.

- Emotional highs and lows are bound to be natural consequences of having faced your mortality and they may take some time to run their course. That's okay.

- You are not alone in feeling how you do. Many others who have faced cancer have felt this way.

- Life is about choice more than chance — you have the power to work to influence every aspect of your life.

- Fear is a lifelong companion for everyone, but is not an obstacle to anything, including living an incredibly good life.

- No matter what challenges are in your life, there is always much to be grateful for. You have survived a significant ordeal and now have a second chance on life!

Actions

- Review lifestyle habits — diet, sleep and exercise in particular — to ensure you are allowing body to support mind and spirit.

- Meditate regularly.

- Join, or if necessary start, a cancer survivors' support group and share your concerns and experiences with the members.

- Talk to your loved ones about how you feel, and listen to how they feel. As difficult as it may be, help them understand how your experience has affected you. If possible, ease their concerns.

- If necessary, seek the assistance of a trained counsellor or psychologist to talk through your feelings. Involve your spouse/partner so that you both gain understanding and healing.

- Apply visualisation, affirmations and positive language use to your cause, paying heed to this advice:

  Be careful of your thoughts, for your thoughts become your words.
  Be careful of your words, for your words become your actions.
  Be careful of your actions, for your actions become your habits.
  Be careful of your habits, for your habits become your character.
  Be careful of your character, for your character becomes your destiny.

- Work through the life path audit (outlined in chapter 13). Review needs and wants to ensure you move closer to your own way of being, relating and creating.

- Use laughter as therapy — create opportunities to laugh with your spouse and loved ones to ease tensions and strengthen bonds.

- Write about your feelings and experiences to help express and release anxieties and despondency.

- Engage in other creative pursuits that appeal to you.

- Use music as therapy.

- Give back. Consider using your experiences to help others going through what you have, in whatever way appeals to you.

- Read and re-read the following chapter. It offers insights, hope and optimism about the significant life-enhancing benefits that can be realised from your experiences.

Your search for closure from the cancer diagnosis and battle that followed may take more time than you expected and might involve various changes in your life. This does not happen for all cancer survivors and when it does, ultimately it may not be a bad thing. While the process of cancer survivorship is sometimes not an easy one, like all journeys of self-discovery, the rewards can be amazing. I discuss this in the next and final chapter.

18

A life with new meaning

As you contemplate your life after cancer, take solace from the fact that for all the challenges you may have after your treatments cease, there are more corresponding benefits if you choose to recognise and realise them. Many if not most cancer survivors ultimately feel their brush with mortality was a blessing in disguise.

Important lessons come from a cancer encounter, including two pearls: the true value of time, and the antidote effect that taking action has on fear.

You've also had the opportunity to take stock of what and who you hold most dearly in life, to assess where you might not have honoured them in the way you would have wanted to and to use the second chance you've worked for to change your behaviours and to right the wrongs.

And with the extreme reality check you've had, you may find yourself re-entering life re-born, intent on making the most out of every day and on creating a life full of meaning.

This final chapter discusses these important points and endeavours to inspire you into action as you embark on the next stage of your life's journey.

Action conquers fear!

As if to compensate you for the suffering and anguish you have had to contend with, your cancer battle has provided you with a gift that will serve you well for the rest of your life: the ability to overcome the two biggest impediments to human endeavour — fear and procrastination.

Where in the past you might have allowed fear to hold you back from what you most wanted to do, create or pursue, your cancer encounter has shown you the reserves of strength and resilience you have at your disposal. Having coped with and prevailed through the most trying circumstances of your life, you know that fear can't stop you doing, creating or pursuing anything you want to.

Procrastination has curtailed many people's dreams and ambitions. It can be born out of fear, but often stems from the mistaken idea that there is unlimited time to achieve what we want to. Truly understanding *now* time is life itself and a limited commodity, will give a healthier respect for what you do with it. You will recognise the madness of waiting until some specified 'whens-day' (*when* you retire; *when* your mortgage is paid off; *when* your children have left home; *when* your stars align) before you embark on the life you would most want to live.

Dr Susan Jeffers, author of the world-famous *Feel the Fear and Do It Anyway* and cancer survivor, has helped millions to face their fears and overcome procrastination. I asked her for her view on coping with fear, and life after cancer:

> My own experience with breast cancer many years ago showed me that you can create something good out of anything...even cancer. I chose (and it is a choice) not to be a victim ('poor me!'); instead, I chose to be a winner as I looked for and found all the good that can come from something as difficult and frightening as cancer. And the phrase I devised to keep me confident throughout, and it still keeps me in good stead, was "Whatever happens, I'll handle it." You will notice that as you keep repeating this affirmation to yourself over and over again, you realise that you really can handle it all. You can learn from it...you can grow from it...you can help the world in your own special way. Yes, you can handle it all.

With the knowledge that you can handle anything life puts to you, and that postponing life is a strategy fraught with risk, you will hopefully choose to live each day from now on boldly and fully.

Making up for lost time

It has been said the greatest danger for most of us is not that our aim in life is too high and we miss it, but that we aim too low and hit it. Many people retain low expectations of life and realise them. Others seem to be aiming high, but have embarked on career and life paths contrary to their heart-felt choice to accommodate the expectations of others, because it seemed more socially acceptable to do so, or simply because it appeared to be an easier way to go.

The consequence of all these choices can be a life void of adventure, passion and wonder, leading to ambivalence about life or worse, soul sickness involving depression, despondency and hopelessness.

what cancer could do to my physical body, living without meaning did to my mind and soul

I have experienced this all-too-common scenario. I found that what cancer could do to my physical body, living without meaning did to my mind and soul. The cost of not taking chances was far higher than the initial discomfort when I took them. As I increasingly dared to go with my heart, setting caution to the wind and pursuing goals that aligned with my ambitions *and* my passions, I found meaning at every turn and my life improved exponentially.

As the saying goes, *some people change their ways when they see the light, others when they feel the heat*. You now have both light and heat to call on to help you make any changes you need in your life. You have a process (chapter 13) to develop an inspiring vision for the future, which — when given wings by courage — will serve as your light, drawing you into a life with greater meaning. The regrets you had about missed opportunities and ill-conceived priorities create pain. Use that as the heat, to *push* you towards life.

Chances are you lamented some or all of the following during your battle:

1. How fast time had gone by.

2. Missed opportunities in life — dreams held but not pursued or abandoned prematurely.

3. Not having been more adventurous and free-spirited in your life.

4. Not having involved yourself in life to the extent you would have wanted.

5. That life seemed to take control of you rather than you controlling it, perhaps resulting in a life direction you wouldn't have chosen.

6. Not having appreciated what you'd had enough.

7. Taking things more seriously than you needed to.

8. Uncertainty over the meaning of your life to that point.

9. A smaller suite of achievements than you would have wanted, with questions over what you might have achieved if you'd taken a different path or had exercised more courage.

10. Having taken those you most loved for granted; wishing you'd spent more time with them rather than at work, had more patience with them than you did and taken a greater interest in their needs.

If, like many people, your most heartfelt regret is how you undervalued those closest to you, you now have a chance to atone. A search for meaning need not and should not be an individual pursuit — loving, caring and sharing with others brings richness that little else can. Re-integrating into the world in a way that enables you to develop healthier relationships, gain a sense of control and establish a happier state of mind will ensure you have a good foundation. One that allows you to review and adjust from so that all those things that are important to you are not lost. Your age is not a factor in pursuing this course of action; it is *never* too late to change direction or behaviours to improve the quality of your life.

To design a life with increased meaning, two processes may particularly help. Make a list of those regrets you reflected on or expressed while battling cancer. It will point to what and who you hold most important and what unrealised needs, hopes and dreams you have. The life path audit of chapter 13 provides a simple, effective framework for building on this list. These two actions will determine what holds most meaning for you, what is no longer relevant and how you might bring about changes to create the kind of life you want.

> *a search for meaning need not and should not be an individual pursuit*

Highly creative, successful and fulfilled people live as fully as possible in the present *while* targeting future-based dreams, goals and aspirations. Pursuing a vision for the future as prescribed in chapter 13 shouldn't stop you from taking time to smell the roses along the way. The journey is to be enjoyed. Most benefits are realised on the way to the destination, not on arrival.

Whatever path you choose after surviving cancer, embark on it with a better sense of yourself and a greater depth of character. Your encounter has made you more genuine — more *real* as I like to term it. A story by a cancer survivor who learned through her battle with cancer what it was for her to become *real,* follows. Written in 1995 for a study by Dr Karen

Hassey Dow, and Dr Betty R. Ferrell, this story appeared in an article, 'Portraits of Cancer Survivorship' in the March/April 1996 issue of *Cancer Practice* (Blackwell Publishing):

Becoming Real

There is a classic story by Marjorie Williams entitled, *The Velveteen Rabbit*… the story of how a child's love turns a toy into a real live bunny. But the meaning of the story goes much deeper than that for me…

In 1992, I was diagnosed with inoperable lymphoma. I was 21 years old… I was married two months earlier and you can imagine how devastating the diagnosis was to each of us. To complicate things even further I was five months pregnant at the time. I was told that I needed to have an immediate abortion, and start aggressive chemotherapy right away.

I cannot explain what it was within me that would not allow the abortion to take place. So when the doctors told me that I had to have the abortion, I shook my head 'no' and said that I could not, even though it meant surmounting six weeks of tremendous pain until they could safely remove her from inside me.

The next six weeks were a living nightmare. It is hard to describe in words. I knew that a monster was alive and growing inside me, and for the sake of my baby I did nothing about it. I never took pain medications, for you see I had already undergone anaesthesia twice and knowing what harm I might already have brought to my daughter literally broke my heart, and I was not about to put her in jeopardy again. To complicate things even further, my diagnosis of cancer had a tremendous effect on my marriage.

I did not hold my daughter after her birth as most mothers do… I remember asking if she was all right, but when I was told she was, I closed my eyes and was filled with peace, and I said to myself, "All right God, I can die now." But I didn't die. I awoke from the surgery in terrible pain, but very much alive.

For five days I didn't hold my baby. On each of those five days I would wander down to the nursery and place my hand over the little plastic tent that she lay under. I would stand there for hours, until one of the nurses demanded that I rest. I would stand there and cry, longing to take my baby in my arms, and to feel like a real mother. I wanted to tell her that I had fought for her life for so long and that now I was fighting for my own.

I underwent a CAT scan that revealed tumours all along my aortic vein. My prognosis was guarded. I received my first dose of chemotherapy.

The baby and I were released from the hospital to hospice care. I was left feeling very alone and confused for I had been told of my prognosis, and told that I might not have much time left.

I continued with treatments, receiving them every three weeks, for eight long months. During the course of them, I lost my hair, my beauty, my pride, and my husband. He said, "I no longer find you attractive, you have too many scars and not enough hair." My daughter and I have not seen him since.

That night I tucked my baby in her crib again, and before I closed the door I noticed that one of her books had fallen from its place on the shelf. Instead of replacing it, I carried it with me to the living room, sat down in a chair by the fire, and began reading *The Velveteen Rabbit*.

"What's Real?" asked the rabbit one day as he and the skin horse were laying side by side near the nursery. "Does it mean having things that buzz inside you and a stick-out handle?"

"Real isn't how you're made," said the skin horse, "It is something that happens to you, when a child loves you for a long, long time, not just to play with, but REALLY loves you, then you become Real."

"Does it hurt?" asked the rabbit.

"Sometimes," said the skin horse, "but when you're Real you don't mind being hurt."

"Does it happen all at once, or bit by bit?" asked the rabbit.

"It doesn't happen all at once," said the skin horse. "You become. It takes a long time. That's why it doesn't often happen to people who break easily, or who have to be carefully kept. Generally, by the time you are Real, most of your hair has been loved off and your eyes drop out and you get loose in the joints and very shabby. But these things don't matter because once you are Real, you cannot be ugly, except to people who don't understand."

When I entered the treatment room to receive my last dose of chemotherapy, I bowed my head in a silent prayer for to me this had become a holy place, no less holy than a church or temple. For it was here that I learned all that there is to know about life. It was here that I learned how to live. I learned about Real love. I learned about Real pain and I learned how Real happiness is achieved.

Sometimes it takes difficulties to make us better, strong people. But most of all, I learned that I am very, very Real. I am in complete remission now. I also had the pleasure of sharing my daughter's first birthday with her, a day I thought I would never see. My goal for a time was to live long enough for her to remember me. Now I am certain I will live long enough to meet my grandchildren.

"There is just one life for each of us: our own" — Euripides

As you emerge as a cancer survivor, you know you are *real*. In the darkest hours of your life you have received the care and support of your family and your friends: so you know you are loved. You were nurtured and tended to with care, concern and compassion by your medical team and by many others in the hospital: so you know that you matter to others too. You discovered what being 'a fighter' really means and you took action time and again to support your recovery cause despite your fears, your pain and your suffering: so you know you are courageous and resilient. You have cared for the recovery of others fighting for their lives too. You felt for them, sometimes cried for them, hoped or prayed for them: so you know you are compassionate and loving.

For as long as you live you now have everything you might need to cope with your post-treatment challenges and to pursue a life of real meaning that honours you as the unique individual you are. The path you take is yours to choose, but my plea is to reach high and follow your heart. I wish you much life and much happiness!

Further recommended reading

Cousins, N (1979). *Anatomy of an Illness*
New York: WW Norton & Co.

Jeffers, S (1987). *Feel the Fear and Do It Anyway*
London: Century Hutchison Ltd

Kane, J (2001). *How to Heal: a guide for caregivers*
New York: Helios Press

LeShan, L (1980). *You Can Fight for Your Life*
USA: M Evans & Co

Little, M, Sayers, E-J, Paul, K (2001). *Surviving Survival: life after cancer*
Marrickville, Australia: Choice Books

Ritberger, C (2000). *What Color is Your Personality?*
Carlsbad, CA: Hay House, Inc, Publishers

Index

Contacting Phil

Phil Kerslake welcomes contact to:

- Share your feelings about this book or your experiences in adopting its methods

- Ask about his speaking services

- Invite him to present to a forum on aspects of the book

- Request media interviews or other media involvement

- Seek consent to cite or reproduce material from this book

email: phil@LifePaths.co.nz

PO Box 13 853, Johnsonville, Wellington 6440, New Zealand